Corneal Disease

Thomas Reinhard • Frank Larkin
Editors

Corneal Disease

Recent Developments in Diagnosis and Therapy

Springer

Editors
Prof. Dr. med. Thomas Reinhard
University Eye Hospital
Freiburg
Germany

Dr. Frank Larkin
Moorfields Eye Hospital
London
UK

ISBN 978-3-642-28746-6 ISBN 978-3-642-28747-3 (eBook)
DOI 10.1007/978-3-642-28747-3
Springer Heidelberg New York Dordrecht London

Library of Congress Control Number: 2012943838

Printed on acid-free paper

Springer is part of Springer Science+Business Media (www.springer.com)

Preface

In this edition we have gathered a number of chapters on diagnosis and management of corneal disorders.

Miller, Girgis, Karp and Alfonso discuss mycobacterial keratitis, uncommon but increasingly encountered following ocular surgery or trauma. Diagnosis and medical therapy remain challenging for this infection.

Sueke, Horsburgh, Gilbert, Shankar, Neal and Kaye present a pragmatic approach to antibacterial chemotherapy in keratitis. Corneal specialists working in referral clinics will be particularly interested in their forward look to new antibacterial agents.

While familial keratoconus is very uncommon in Europe and North America, there is an increasing interest in information we can discover on keratoconus pathogenesis from apparently unaffected relatives with subclinical ectasia signs. Willoughby and Lechner review their own work and the recent published literature.

Imaging techniques have become a valuable component in diagnosis of corneal diseases, ranging from infections to corneal dystrophies. Labbé, Denoyer and Baudouin further show that confocal microscopy and ocular coherence tomography may facilitate clinical follow-up after corneal surgery.

Cursiefen and Bock discriminate between haem- and lymph-angiogenesis. They demonstrate that novel anti-angiogenic agents directed at blood or lymph vessels can significantly improve allograft survival by regression of corneal vessels pre- as well as post- transplantation.

For keratoplasty it is vital that corneal surgeons have access to cornea banks with robust and effective quality and risk management systems. Pels and Pollock illustrate that this is especially true in respect to the increasing practice of eye bank preparation of donor posterior lamellar cornea for endothelial keratoplasty procedures.

Few corneal surgeons undertake corneal transplantation in infants with any regularity. Surgical technical and post-operative management challenges in this transplant recipient group are very different to older patients, as Kim and Rootman describe. We expect that David Rootman's comparatively huge experience in infant keratoplasty will be a useful reference to those readers faced with occasional infant candidates for surgery.

We hope you enjoy reading this book.

Thomas Reinhard
Frank Larkin

Contents

Contributors

Eduardo C. Alfonso, M.D. Department of Ophthalmology, University of Miami Miller School of Medicine, Miami, USA

Christophe Baudouin, M.D., Ph.D. Department of Ophthalmology III, Quinze-Vingts National Ophthalmology Hospital, Paris, France

Felix Bock Department of Ophthalmology, University of Cologne, Köln, Germany

Claus Cursiefen, M.D., FEBO Department of Ophthalmology, University of Cologne, Köln, Germany

Alexandre Denoyer, M.D. Department of Ophthalmology III, Quinze-Vingts National Ophthalmology Hospital, Paris, France

R. Gilbert St. Paul's Eye Unit, Royal Liverpool University Hospital, 8Z Link, Liverpool, UK

Dalia Girgis, M.D. Department of Ophthalmology, University of Miami Miller School of Medicine, Miami, USA

M. Horsburgh Institute of Integrative Biology, University of Liverpool, Liverpool, UK

Carol Karp, M.D. Department of Ophthalmology, University of Miami Miller School of Medicine, Miami, USA

Stephen B. Kaye St. Paul's Eye Unit, Royal Liverpool University Hospital, 8Z Link, Liverpool, UK

Peter Kim, MBBS (Hons), FRANZCO Department of Ophthalmology, Toronto Western Hospital, University of Toronto, Toronto, ON, Canada

Antoine Labbé, M.D., Ph.D. Department of Ophthalmology III, Quinze-Vingts National Ophthalmology Hospital, Paris, France

Judith Lechner School of Medicine, Dentistry and Biomedical Sciences, Centre for Vision and Vascular Science, Queen's University Belfast, Royal Victoria Hospital, Belfast, UK

Darlene Miller, DHSc. Department of Ophthalmology, University of Miami Miller School of Medicine, Miami, USA

T.J. Neal Department of Microbiology, Royal Liverpool University Hospital, Liverpool, UK

Elisabeth Pels, Ph.D. Cornea Bank Amsterdam, Euro Tissue Bank, Beverwijk, The Netherlands

Graeme Pollock, Ph.D. Lions Eye Donation Service Melbourne, Royal Victorian Eye and Ear Hospital, Melbourne, VIC, Australia

David S. Rootman, M.D., FRCSC Department of Ophthalmology and Visual Sciences, Toronto Western Hospital, University of Toronto, Toronto, ON, Canada

J. Shankar St. Paul's Eye Unit, Royal Liverpool University Hospital, 8Z Link, Liverpool, UK

H. Sueke St. Paul's Eye Unit, Royal Liverpool University Hospital, 8Z Link, Liverpool, UK

Colin E. Willoughby School of Medicine, Dentistry and Biomedical Sciences, Centre for Vision and Vascular Science, Queen's University Belfast, Royal Victoria Hospital, Belfast, UK

New Aspects in the Diagnosis and Therapy of Mycobacterial Keratitis

1

Darlene Miller, Dalia Girgis, Carol Karp, and Eduardo C. Alfonso

Core Messages

- Mycobacterial keratitis is a rare but sight-threatening infection caused by both slow growing (Runyoun Groups I-III) and rapid growing (Runyoun Group IV) members of the genus Mycobacterium following trauma or ocular surgery.
- Mycobacteria are aerobic, nonmotile, nonspore-forming bacilli, ubiquitous in nature and difficult to eradicate with common disinfectants and topical antimicrobials due to the high lipid content of their cell walls.
- Delay in clinical and laboratory diagnosis and confirmation contributes to the protracted clinical course associated with the disease.
- Medical therapy and management remain a challenge.
- Surgical intervention is often required to cure and control the disease.

Mycobacterial keratitis is a rare event [1]. In general, infection rates constitute less than 2% of reported infectious microbial keratitis cases [2, 3]. Rates may vary by geographical locations and have been as high as 8% in some reported series from Asia (Reddy, Lalthia, Huang). Trends in recovery of mycobacteria from keratitis increased in number and diversity in the last decade (Fig. 1.1 and Table 1.1). Disease recognition, confirmation and management, however, remain challenging. Clinical diagnosis is problematic due to delay in presentation, low index of suspicion, mimicry of fungal or viral keratitis, and prior antibiotic and/or corticosteroid therapy. Traditional risk factors have included trauma with metal objects, soil and/or

D. Miller, DHSc. • D. Girgis, M.D. (✉) • C. Karp, M.D. • E.C. Alfonso, M.D.
Department of Ophthalmology, University of Miami Miller School of Medicine, 900 N.W., 17th Street, Miami 33136, USA
e-mail: dmiller@med.miami.edu; dgirgis@uwhealth.org; ckarp@med.miami.edu; ealfonso@med.miami.edu

T. Reinhard, F. Larkin (eds.), *Corneal Disease*,
DOI 10.1007/978-3-642-28747-3_1,

vegetable matter or following surgical interventions such as radial keratotomy, photorefractive keratectomy, cataract surgery, or contact lens wear (Fig. 1.2). Current and emerging risk factors are mainly health care related and include surgical procedures (LASIK, LASEK, DSEK), smart plugs, and other biomaterials (Fig. 1.3). In several patients, no identifiable risk factor has been documented [4–7].

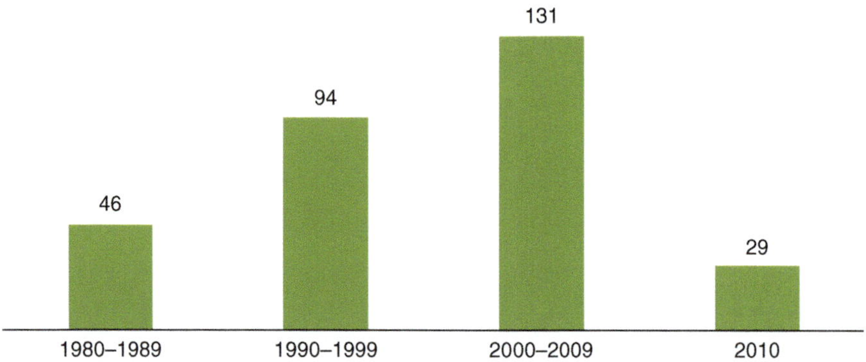

Fig. 1.1 Trends in mycobacterial keratitis cases (literature)

Table 1.1 Frequency and diversity of mycobacterial species recovered from keratitis (published reports 1980–2010), $N=300$

Mycobacteria classification	Sample source		Isolates	
Runyon group	LASIK flap, cornea bed	Non-LASIK scrapings, biopsy	# of isolates	% of isolates
Group I – Photochromogens (Slow growing >7 days for colonies to appear on solid media after subculture; pigment upon light exposure)				
M. asiaticum		1	1	0.33
M. marinum		1	1	0.33
Total	0	2	2	0.66
Group II – Scotochromogens (Slow growing-pigment in dark or light)				
M. flavescens		1	1	0.33
M. gordonae	2	3	5	1.67
M. szulgai	7	1	8	2.67
Total	9	5	14	4.67
Group III – Nonchromogens (Slow growing; nonpigmented)				
M. avium complex	0	2	2	0.67
M. nonchromogenicum	0	1	1	0.33
M. terrae	1		1	0.33
M. triviale	0	1	1	0.33
Total	1	4	5	1.67

Table 1.1 (continued)

Mycobacteria classification	Sample source		Isolates	
Runyon group	LASIK flap, cornea bed	Non-LASIK scrapings, biopsy	# of isolates	% of isolates
Group IV – Rapid Growers (<7 days for colonies to appear on solid media after subculture)				
M. abscessus	7	15	22	7.33
M. chelonae	37	123	130	53.33
M. fortuitum	4	38	42	14.00
M. immunogenum	5	0	5	1.67
M. immnogenum	2	0	2	0.67
M. smegmatis	0	1	1	0.33
Total	55	177	232	77.33
Nontuberculosis Mycobacteria, not otherwise speciated (NTM, NOS)	*5*	*42*	*47*	*15.67*
Total isolates	70	230	300	
% of isolates	23.33	76.67		

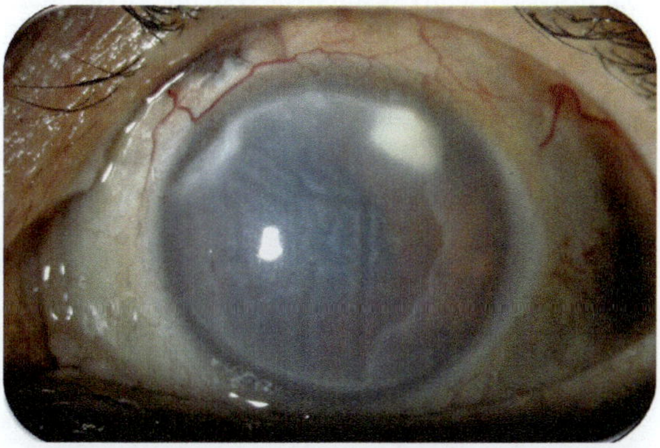

Fig. 1.2 *M. chelonae* mycobacteria following CE/IOL/trabectomy

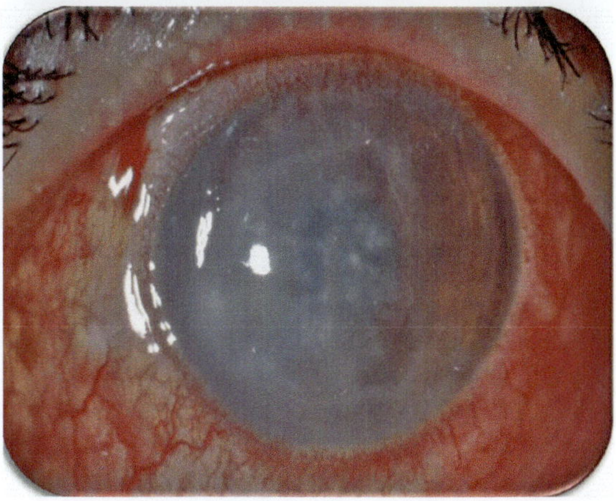

Fig. 1.3 Post LASIK *Mycobacteria abscessus* keratitis

Laboratory confirmation is hindered by delay in culturing, prior therapy, quality and quantity of specimen, inexperienced personnel, and microbial growth rate [1, 3, 7]. Lack of simple, rapid, and accurate methods also adds to the delay in laboratory identification and confirmation.

Organisms

Among the more than 100 mycobacterial species, less than 20 have been associated with microbial keratitis (Table 1.1) [8, 9]. A minimal of 300 cases of mycobacterial keratitis have been reported since the first case by Turner and Stinson in 1965. Nontuberculous species (NTM), also referred to as "atypical mycobacteria" or mycobacteria other than tuberculosis (MOTT) are the most common. The majority of these continue to be rapidly growing, saprophytic species with diverse environmental reservoirs including fresh, salt, and recreational waters, soil, animals and healthy colonized human. Members of the *Mycobacteria chelonae complex* (Runyoun Group IV) have been the most frequent pathogens, constituting 63% and 60% of LASIK and traumatic inoculation cases, respectively (Table 1.1).

True pathogens *M. tuberculosis* and *M. leprae* can directly invade corneal tissue but disease usually results via systemic dissemination or accidental direct inoculation. Less than 5% of patients with *M. tuberculosis* will develop keratitis [10–12]. The clinical presentation is usually an allergic reaction. The numbers are a little higher for patients suffering from leprosy due to direct corneal invasion and ulceration associated with corneal anesthesia [13]. Although rare, these pathogens cause significant morbidity and mortality in endemic areas and are increasingly encountered in the rising population of HIV patients [14].

Nontuberculous species are ubiquitous in nature and resistant to traditional mycobacterial drugs as well as chlorine and other disinfectants. Increasingly, sporadic single cases or outbreaks are associated with unusually or slow growing mycobacteria such as *M. skulgai*, *M. immunogenum*, and/or *M. terrae*. The Runyon classification with modifications is still used to characterize these infections. The classification of isolates is based on the time it takes for colonies to appear on solid media from a subculture rather than growth from clinical samples. Common rapid growers (*M. abscessus*, *M. chelonae*, *M. fortuitum*) usually grow from subculture within 3–7 days while growth after subculture for the slower growers taking up to 8 weeks. All four Runyon groups have been associated with microbial keratitis.

Detection

Conventional techniques for the identification of mycobacterial species employ a battery of phenotypic (growth rate, colony morphology) characteristics and biochemical tests. These are time consuming, labor intensive, expensive, and often inconclusive. The delay in laboratory recovery and identification may impede clinical diagnosis [2, 15–17]. An updated algorithm using molecular and traditional

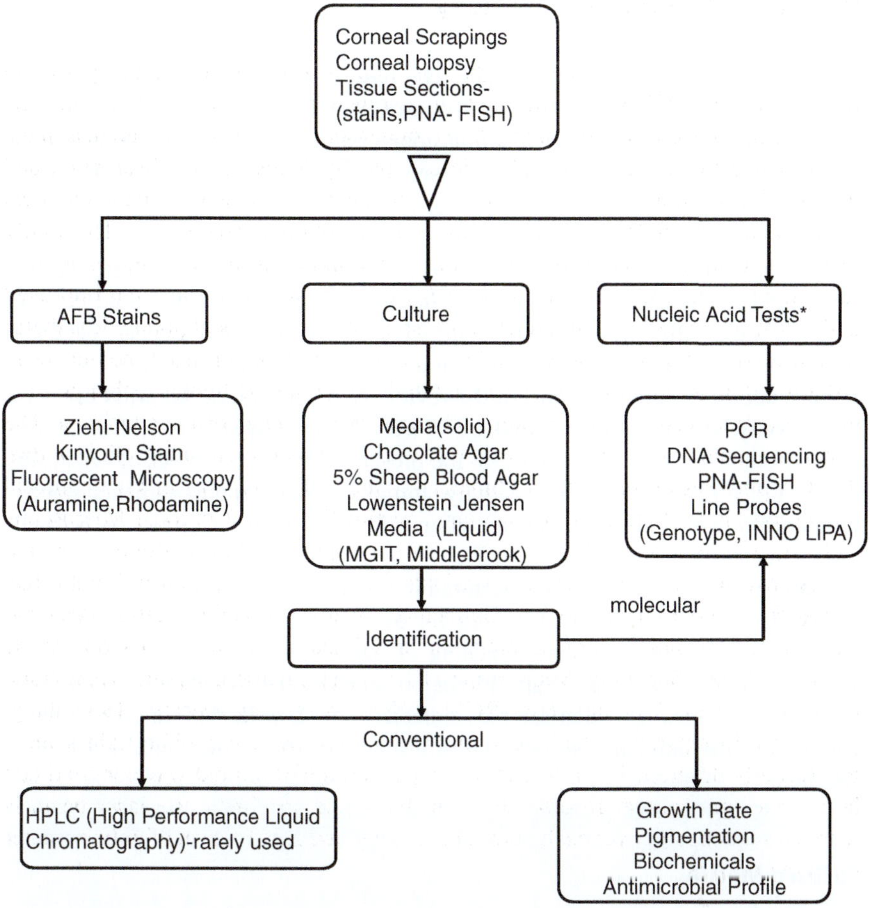

Fig. 1.4 Algorithm for mycobacterial keratitis detection and identification

methods for recovery and identification of mycobacterial species associated with mycobacterial keratitis is outlined in Fig. 1.4. Sample size, available services, and laboratory personnel may compromise full implementation of techniques.

New aspects for the detection and identification of mycobacteria in or recovered from ocular samples include use of rapid fluorescent acid fast stains, inoculation of enhanced culture media, and implementation of a variety of nucleic acid-based assays coupled with hybridization procedures and DNA sequencing.

Acid Fast Smears

Acid fast stains and recovery on solid media continue to be the cornerstones for laboratory and clinical confirmation of mycobacterial keratitis. The carbol fuschin-based stains (Kinyoun (cold) and Ziehl Neelsen (hot)) are important tools in the rapid and direct detection of acid fast bacilli in corneal scrapings, biopsies, and material collected from under the LASIK flap. The basic stain includes flooding a heat-fixed slide with carbol fuschin for 3–5 min, decolorization with acid alcohol, wash step, and application of a 1-min counterstain. A modified Kinyoun stain using a weaker decolorizer may be more sensitive for confirming the rapidly growing mycobacteria due to their wearker or inconsistent staining with the first two preparations (<10%) [9, 18].

Although fluorescent stains (auramine or auramine–rhodamine) are generally more rapid and sensitive than the carbol fuschin stains, many of the rapid growers may not stain with these fluorochromes [9, 18]. In positive smears, acid-fast organisms will appear orange-yellow in a black background or yellow-green in the absence of the counterstain. In the review of mycobacteria keratitis cases by Huang, only 50% of culture positive cases were detected by smear [5]. Limitations of these studies is the requirement for the presence of a high number of organisms ($\geq 10^{3-4}$ CFU/ml) required for positivity. Initial corneal scrapings/smears contain numbers below this threshold and are often acid fast negative. Correlation between smears and culture is poor.

A recent, new modification of the auramine stain, Rapid-Auramine O, (Scientific Device, Inc, Des Plaines, IL) provides for quicker (2 min vs. 22 min) and more sensitive (brighter, less debris) screening of mycobacteria from clinical samples including *M. fortuitum* (100%) and *M. chelonae* (80%) [19]. This might be useful in evaluating or screening ocular samples collected from LASIK flaps or corneal biopsies where the infecting microorganism may be above the stain's detection threshold.

Culture Media

Both liquid and solid media are recommended for optimal recovery and quicker identification of mycobacteria species. The most frequently involved pathogens (the rapid growers) are recovered from corneal scrapings, tissues, or biopsy within 3 days on routine solid media (chocolate, blood agar, Sabouraud agars) and special media (Lowenstein-Jensen and Middlebrook agars) (Figs. 1.5 and 1.6). Dependent on the quality and quantity of sample, initial recovery of mycobacterial species can take up to 10 days.

Slow growers (Runyoun Groups I-III) and *Mycobacterium tuberculosis* grow poorly or not at all on routine laboratory media. Scrapings should be inoculated on to Lowenstein-Jensen, Middlebrook, or Ogawa media for recovery. Recovery rates range from 2 to 8 weeks. Broth media (MGIT, Middlebrook, and Bactec media) have been used to recover mycobacteria from corneal samples. Organisms were recovered on average within 3 days from inoculation. *M. leprae* has not been grown on artificial laboratory media.

A new type of solid media has been developed for the recovery, identification, and susceptibility of mycobacteria species. TK Medium (*M. tuberculosis* complex)

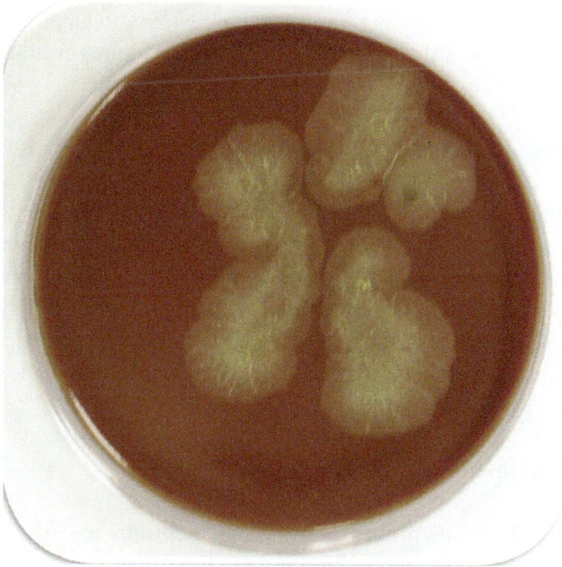

Fig. 1.5 *M. chelonae* – chocolate-day 10

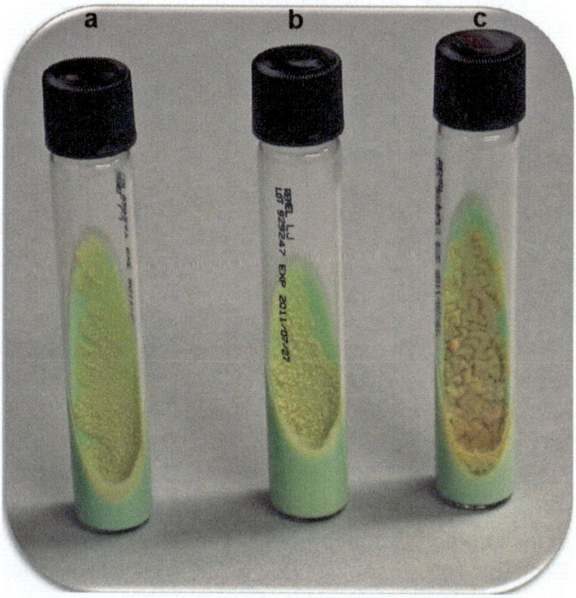

Fig. 1.6 *Mycobacteria* and *Nocardia* species on Lowenstein-Jensen agar (14 day growth). (**a**) *M. avium*-intracellulare, (**b**) *M. fortuitum*, (**c**) *Nocardia asteroides*

and TK PNB (MOTT) allows for rapid identification of mycobacterial species based on colorimetric changes in the media. The color changes are read manually or in an automated system. *Mycobacteria* species can be recovered 5–18 days earlier than with conventional solid media. Antituberculosis drugs have been incorporated into the media for susceptibility testing. No multicenter trials have been conducted evaluating the utility of the media in low, medium, or high prevalence areas [20].

Molecular Tests

Molecular assays based on amplification techniques targeting insertion element IS 6110, 16 S rRNA gene, internal transcribed spacer gene, or the *hsp*65 gene that can detect or confirm the presence of mycobacteria in clinical samples include routine, nested, real-time PCR, and PCR combined with enzyme restriction analysis (PCR-REA). Mycobacteria identification is confirmed by species-specific probes and/or their distinct enzymatic profile or patterns [21, 22].

Nucleic Acid Hybridization Probes

Nucleic acid probes allow rapid identification of select, common mycobacteria species. Probes can be employed for direct detection of mycobacteria in smear positive or highly suspicious tissue samples. Acridinium ester-labeled DNA probes complementary to the16S rRNA mycobacteria gene (AccuProbe; Gen-Probe Inc, San Diego, CA) are available for confirmation of *M. tuberculosis* complex, *M. avium* complex, *M. kansaii*, and *M. gordonae*. Probes are added to sonicated colonies, form a DNA–rRNA hybrid and are detected by a luminometer. Turnaround time is about 2 h. Sensitivity varies depending on the species. Comparison with Bactec, AccuProbes sensitivity was >85–100 and 100% specificity. Turnaround time is 2 h [21, 22].

Line Probes

Several line probe assays have been developed for the detection of mycobacteria species targeting either the 16S-23S rRNA internal spacer region (INNO LiPA Mycobacteria v2, Innogenetics, Ghent, Belgium) or the 23S rRNA gene (GenoType Mycobacteria MTBC, GenoType Mycobacterium CM, GenoType AS, GenoType LepraeDR, Hain Lifescience, Nehren, Germany) [21, 22].

The assays are based on the reverse hybridization of biotinylated PCR products to their complementary probes immobilized as parallel lines on a membrane strip. Detection and identification is via colorimetric detection using an automated instrument. Seventeen of the most frequently encountered mycobacteria species, including *M. tuberculosis* complex, *M. avium*, *M. intracellulare*, *M. chelonae*, *M. gordonae*, *M. smegmatis*, *M. fortuitum* complex, and *M. marinum* are identified with the Inno-LiPA kit, while the combination of the first three Hain Lifescience kits (GenoType MTBC, CM, AS) can identify *M. tuberculosis* and 30 different nontuberculous mycobacteria including the most frequently species isolated from mycobacterial keratitis. Colonies growing on solid or liquid media can be used with these two systems. Turnaround time is 6 h. The *M. leprae* kit can confirm the presence of *M. leprae* as well as resistance to dapsone, ofloxacin, and rifampicin [21, 22].

DNA Sequencing

DNA sequencing is considered the "gold standard" for definitive identification of mycobacteria species. The procedure includes amplification with universal mycobacterial primers (6S rRNA gene or the *hsp65* gene) followed by product (DNA) sequencing in an automated sequencer. Sequences are then compared with a database with known mycobacteria sequences [21, 22].

FISH (Fluorescent In Situ Hybridization) Assay

PNA-FISH-Fluorescent in situ hybridization tests using peptide nucleic acid coupled to a fluorescent probe are available for the detection of *Mycobacteria tuberculosis, M. leprae*, and nontuberculous mycobacteria from clinical samples, cultures, tissues, and paraffin sections [23]. It is a rapid and accurate technique for species identification and direct detection in tissues [24].

DNA Microarray

Hybridization of species-specific probes on a DNA chip allows for rapid identification of M. tuberculosis and other mycobacteria species. This technique is currently restricted to reference or research laboratories. Due to expense, this technique is currently restricted to reference or research laboratories [21, 22].

Pyrosequencing technology is a unique technique based on nucleic acid sequencing by addition and detection of released pyrophosphate during synthesis [25]. Tuohy et al. used it as a tool for the identification of mycobacterial species and documented it as a rapid and acceptable method for identifying the most frequent mycobacterial species recovered from clinical samples. Galor et al. used it to identify a case of Nocardia keratitis [26]. It could provide a rapid method for identification of unusual ocular pathogens including mycobacteria species [25].

Pulse Field Gel Electrophoresis (PFGE)

Pulse field gel electrophoresis is a molecular typing method that can characterize mycobacterial species associated with outbreaks. It has been instrumental in confirming LASIK outbreaks in the United States and Brazil [4, 27, 28]. It is time-consuming and requires molecular expertise.

The polymerase chain reaction and other molecular diagnostics are ideal for the detection and/or confirmation of mycobacteria species in ocular samples due to limited sample, prior therapy, delay in presentation, and laboratory studies. Several authors have used these techniques to detect and identify ocular mycobacterial isolates. They afford a more rapid and sensitive method for recovery and identification for both culture-negative and culture-positive samples [29–36].

Management

Clinical Diagnosis

Delay in clinical diagnosis is a common problem in the management of mycobacterial keratitis. The delay in diagnosis contributes to the protracted course and poor patient outcomes. Recognizing the clinical signs of mycobacterial keratitis is crucial in improving the clinical diagnosis. This can be difficult because of the chronic, indolent, progression of the disease, delay in presentation, prior use of steroids and topical antibiotics, mimicry of herpetic, fungal or diffuse lamellar keratitis, and lack of rapid, routine laboratory studies [1, 3, 6, 7, 15].

Clues for patients presenting with postLASIK infections include delayed onset, nonresponsive to topical antibiotics, presence of a white infiltrate in the corneal interface with spread to posterior stromal with or without satellite lesions, and tissue necrosis [1, 3–6, 33, 37–39].

Risk factors for patients with non-LASIK associated mycobacterial keratitis include corneal foreign body, trauma, contact lens wear, penetrating keratoplasty, cataract surgery, corneal suture, radial keratotomy, and chronic steroid use [3, 36]. More than 50% of patients with non-LASIK associated keratitis have an antecedent history of trauma or corneal surgery.

Medical Therapy

Minimal progress in the treatment and management of mycobacterial keratitis has been made since the first case diagnosed by Turner and Stinson. No standard or ideal antibiotic regimen for the prevention or treatment of mycobacterial keratitis exists. A variety of drugs including macrolides (azithromycin, clarithromycin), fluoroquinolones (ciprofloxacin, levofloxacin, gatifloxacin, and moxifloxacin), and aminoglycosides (amikacin, gentamicin, kanamycin, tobramycin) have been used with mixed results [3, 4, 15, 27–29, 40]. Both in vivo and in vitro responses to the commonly used antibiotics are variable and species specific [41] (Table 1.2). In vitro susceptibility results and in vivo response may also differ by source and geographical region [3, 42–47]) Correlation between the two is quite poor and frequently unreliable.

Contributing to this discord is the high lipid content of the organism's cell wall, poor drug penetration, slow growth rate of the organism, drug toxicity, biofilm formation, and lack of simple, accurate methods for susceptibility testing.

A summary of in vitro results from our Institute (ocular) and the literature (ocular and nonocular) is highlighted in Fig. 1.7 and Table 1.2. Rates for the aminoglycosides

Table 1.2 Antimicrobial activity of common keratitis isolates

Antimicrobial[a]	90% susceptible	≤90% susceptible
Amikacin	*M. abscessus, M. chelonae, M. mucogenicum, M. fortuitum*	
Tobramycin	*M. abscessus*	*M. chelonae, M. fortuitum*
Azithromycin	*M. abscessus, M. chelonae*	*M. fortuitum*
Clarithromycin	*M. abscessus, M. chelonae*	*M. fortuitum*
Ciprofloxacin	*M. fortuitum*	*M. abscessus, M. chelonae, M. immnogenum*
Levofloxacin	*M. fortuitum, M. tuberculosis, M. leprae*	*M. abscessus, M. cheloane*
Gatifloxacin	*M. fortuitum, M. tuberculosis, M. leprae*	*M. abscessus, M. cheloane*
Moxifloxacin	*M. fortuitum, M. tuberculosis, M. leprae*	*M. abscessus, M. cheloane*
Linezolid	*M. tuberculosis, M. fortuitum, M. smegmatis, M. chelonae*	*M. abscessus*

[a]References Brown-Elliot, Wallace, Reddy, Ford, Griffith for ATM

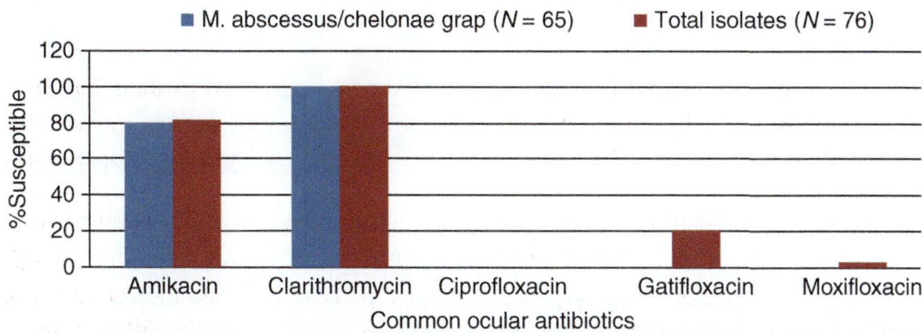

Fig. 1.7 In vitro susceptibility of BPEI mycobacterial keratitis isolates

ranged from 82% to 100%, with *M. chelonae and M. fortuitum* more susceptible in vitro to amikacin. *M. fortuitum* was more susceptible to the fluoroquinolones than was *M. abscessus* or *M. chelonae*, while the latter two were more susceptible to the macrolides. High-level resistance among rapidly growing mycobacteria isolates from Taiwan (<90% susceptible; *M. abscessus* – $N=92$, *M. chelonae* – $N=39$, and *M. fortuitum* group – $N=69$) was reported for fluoroquinolones, macrolides, and tobramycin. All isolates were susceptible to amikacin. None of the isolates were recovered from keratitis [48]. Both clinical failure and high-level resistance to the fluoroquinolones, including gatifloxacin and moxifloxacin were documented for *M. chelonae* isolates recovered from a LASIK outbreak [4, 15, 49, 50].

Current recommendations for the management of mycobacteria keratitis include aggressive, topical combination therapy with clarithromycin (10 mg/ml) or azithromycin (2 mg/ml) supplemented with amikacin (50 mg/ml) or a fourth-generation fluoroquinolone [5, 6, 51]. Ford et al. documented clinical failure in 60% of their patients treated with the two-drug regimen of amikacin and clarithromycin, despite being susceptible in vitro [3]. Others documented similar rates of clinical failure with the two-drug regimen [15, 16, 40, 52–54]. The majority of patients (70%) with

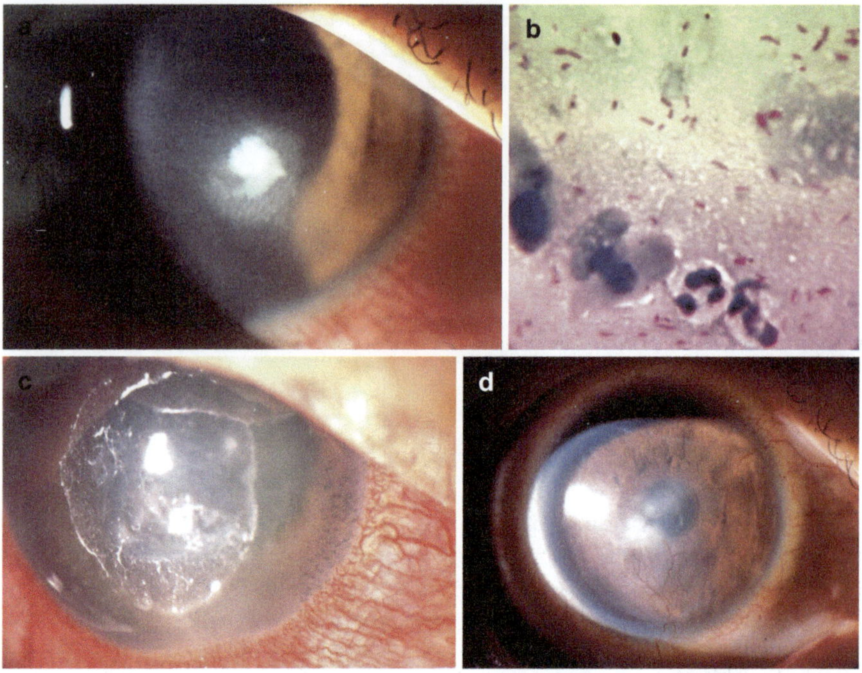

Fig. 1.8 A 31-year old woman presented with a central interface infiltrate in her right eye 7 weeks after LASIK (**a**). Multiple acid-fast bacilli, epithelial cells and polymorphonuclear leukocytes were demonstrated from scrapings taken from the infiltrate (**b**). The flap was amputated 3 weeks later as new infiltrates appeared (**c**). Three months after onset, her cornea has a resolving scar with neovascularization, and her vision improved from hand motions to 20/50 (**d**) (From Solomon et al. [1], with permission)

mycobacterial infections following LASIK were managed with regimens of 3 (49%) or 4 (21%) drugs [6]. Successful medical therapy alone is rare. Epithelial debridement or in the case of LASIK, flap amputation is often required to enhance penetration of the medications and debulk the infection (Fig. 1.8).

Hu and colleagues [46, 55] demonstrated in vitro antagonism when an aminoglycoside was combined with imipenem, ciprofloxacin, and/or clarithromycin. This might account for the protracted course and often need to switch antibiotics to achieve successful eradication. Matoba et al. also found indifferent or antagonist results when combining amikacin with ciprofloxacin to treat mycobacterial keratitis [54]. A high rate of treatment failure in nontuberculous pulmonary disease using the combination of amikacin and clarithromycin has also been documented [5, 41].

Prolonged therapy with amikacin can lead to the emergence of resistant isolates. Similarly, the presence of an inducible erythromycin-resistant gene in all *M. fortuitum* isolates can lead to treatment failure with prolonged use of the macrolides to treat mycobacterial keratitis. Selection of clarithromycin-resistant isolates has also been documented with prolonged therapy [41, 43, 56].

Addition of a fluoroquinolone (ciprofloxacin, moxifloxacin, or gatifloxacin) to this regimen has improved epithelial healing and final visual outcome [50].

M. fortuitum and other nontuberculous mycobacteria are more susceptible in vivo and in vitro to the fluoroquinolones than are members of the *M. abscessus–M. chelonae* complex [47, 57, 58] (Table 1.2). Moshifar et al. reported a case of moxifloxacin-resistant *M. chelonae* recovered from a patient on Vigamox for prophylaxis post-LASIK [31]. De la Cruz reported two more cases unresponsive to gatifloxacin in vivo and documented resistance to both moxifloxacin and gatifloxacin in vitro [59].

Few new antibiotics are available for medical therapy or prophylaxis of mycobacterial keratitis. Those that have demonstrated both in vitro and in vivo include linezolid, telithromycin, and tigecycline. Linezolid has been used to treat *M. tuberculosis* and has >90% in vitro efficacy for most rapid growers [60, 61]. Telithromycin, a newer macrolide, had moderate (<90% in vitro efficacy) against the rapid growers and was not effective against *M. tuberculosis* and/or the slow-growing mycobacteria [45, 62]. Tigecycline a new type of tetracycline derivative had in vitro MICs of ≤1 ug/ml for the most common mycobacteria recovered from keratitis [56, 63, 64].

Clofazimine, an antileprosy drug, has been evaluated against rapidly growing mycobacteria with good in vitro results [65, 66]. Shen et al. evaluated clofazimine in vitro against rapidly growing mycobacteria. MIC90 for the most commonly recovered isolates was ≤1ug/ml (range 0.5–1.0 mg/ml). Susceptibility profiles were *M. abscessus* (99.1%, $N=117$), *M. chelonae* (100%, $N=20$), and *M. fortuitum* (91.7%, $N=48$). Synergy with amikacin was documented for all *M. abscessus* and *M. chelonae* isolates and 48% of the *M. fortuitum* isolates. Results in vitro suggest that clofazimine alone or with amikacin may be effective against Group IV mycobacteria species [67]. No clinical data is available. The drug is not available in the United States and WHO discourages its widespread use for treating infections other than leprosy. It has been used as adjunctive therapy to treat *M. avium* complex pulmonary infections [65–67].

Besifloxacin is a new fluoroquinolone with similar or lower MIC90s against common ocular pathogens. No clinical or in vitro data are available for the treatment or in vitro susceptibility of mycobacterial species with this new fluoroquinolone [68, 69].

Corticosteroids should be used with caution in patients confirmed with mycobacterial keratitis. They may mask the disease progression, retard immune response, and accelerate growth and dissemination of the organisms [1, 3, 5–7, 15, 66, 70].

New drug delivery systems using liposomes and nanoparticles to deliver antituberculous drugs are in development. These systems are already used to deliver steroids and antiherpetic drugs to the eye. Mycobacterial keratitis might be an ideal disease to evaluate these two drug delivery systems [8].

Surgical Intervention

Surgical intervention is often necessary to affect a cure and control the progression of disease. Debridement reduces the microbial load which is an essential part of management and cure of mycobacterial keratitis [6, 7, 38, 71]. Huang et al. performed early keratectomy in 15/22 (68%) cases of nontuberculous keratitis

(19-*M. chelonae*, 3-*M. fortuitum*) seen in their hospital over a 3-year period. Surgery was performed on severe and recalcitrant cases which were unresponsive to medical therapy (50 mg/ml of amikacin) [5]. Hu also performed lamellar keratectomy on 7 of 9 patients recalcitrant to medical therapy with amikacin [38]. John and Velotta documented flap removal in 54% of patients in their review of complications of nontuberculous mycobacterial postLASIK [6]. Better patient outcomes are associated with early lifting of the flap, debridement and soaking or irrigating the bed and flap with a macrolide or fourth-generation fluoroquinolone.

Penetrating Keratoplasty

Penetrating keratoplasty may be necessary to manage both LASIK and non-LASIK cases unresponsive to medical therapy. These should be performed on patients with extensive full thickness or those threatening perforation [6, 7, 15]. Susiyanti used deep anterior lamellar keratoplasty (DALK) as an alternative to PRK to manage several recalcitrant postLASIK cases [72].

Corneal Cross-Linking

Corneal cross-linking has been used to treat recalcitrant keratitis with success for fungal and acanthamoeba keratitis. The procedure strengthens the corneal stroma and simultaneously reduces or eliminates microbial load using a combination of riboflavin and UV light [73]. This technique has been used successfully to treat a case of *E. coli* keratitis [74]. To date, there are no reports of it being successfully used to treat mycobacteria keratitis. It could serve as a possible alternative to PRK or other surgical interventions for unresponsive mycobacteria keratitis. There are some risks associated with the procedure, including secondary bacterial keratitis [75, 76].

Summary for the Clinician

- Diagnosis and management of mycobacterial keratitis remain problematic. Mycobacteria keratitis should be part of the differential diagnosis of any chronic keratitis that does not respond to conventional therapy, especially following trauma or ocular surgery.
- Early clinical recognition, coupled with aggressive combination therapy, prompt laboratory studies, and swift surgical intervention will reduce patient morbidity and result in more favorable clinical outcomes.
- Corticosteroids are counter indicated in the early management of mycobacterial keratitis.
- Evolving molecular techniques are available to help expedite detection, species identification, and clinical diagnosis.

References

1. Solomon A et al (2001) Mycobacterium interface keratitis after laser in situ keratomileusis. Ophthalmology 108(12):2201–2208
2. Daines BS et al (2003) Rapid diagnosis and treatment of mycobacterial keratitis after laser in situ keratomileusis. J Cataract Refract Surg 29(5):1014–1018
3. Ford JG et al (1998) Nontuberculous mycobacterial keratitis in south Florida. Ophthalmology 105(9):1652–1658
4. Freitas D et al (2003) An outbreak of *Mycobacterium chelonae* infection after LASIK. Ophthalmology 110(2):276–285
5. Huang SC et al (1996) Non-tuberculous mycobacterial keratitis: a study of 22 cases. Br J Ophthalmol 80(11):962–968
6. John T, Velotta E (2005) Nontuberculous (atypical) mycobacterial keratitis after LASIK: current status and clinical implications. Cornea 24(3):245–255
7. Karp CL et al (2003) Infectious keratitis after LASIK. Ophthalmology 110(3):503–510
8. Gaspar MM et al (2008) Developments on drug delivery systems for the treatment of mycobacterial infections. Curr Top Med Chem 8(7):579–591
9. Pfyffer GE (2007) Mycobacterium: general characteristics, laboratory detection, and staining procedures. In: Murray PR (ed) Manual of clinical microbiology. ASM Press, Washington, DC
10. Gupta N et al (2008) Necrotizing scleritis and peripheral ulcerative keratitis in a case of Sweet's syndrome found culture-positive for *Mycobacterium tuberculosis*. Ann Trop Med Parasitol 102(6):557–560
11. Zaborowski AG et al (2006) Primary tuberculous keratoconjunctivitis. Eye (Lond) 20(8): 978–979
12. Sheu SJ et al (2001) Ocular manifestations of tuberculosis. Ophthalmology 108(9): 1580–1585
13. John D, Daniel E (1999) Infectious keratitis in leprosy. Br J Ophthalmol 83(2):173–176
14. Trucksis MT, Dunn JM (2010) Mycobacterial diseases of the eye. In: Tasman Q, Jaeger EA (eds) Duane's Ophthalmology on DVD-ROM 2010 edition (foundations of clinical ophthalmology). Lippincott, Williams & Wilkins, New York
15. Biber JM, Kim JY (2011) Nontuberculous mycobacteria keratitis. In: Krachmer JH, Mannis MJ, Holland EJ (eds) Cornea: fundamental, diagnosis and management. Mosby, New York
16. Bullington RH Jr, Lanier JD, Font RL (1992) Nontuberculous mycobacterial keratitis. Report of two cases and review of the literature. Arch Ophthalmol 110(4):519–524
17. Lalitha P, Rathinam SR, Srinivasan M (2004) Ocular infections due to non-tuberculous mycobacteria. Indian J Med Microbiol 22(4):231–237
18. Chapin KC, Lauderdale T (2007) Reagents, stains and media: bacteriology. In: Murray PR (ed) Manual of clinical microbiology. ASM, Washington, DC
19. Hendry C et al (2009) Evaluation of a rapid fluorescent staining method for detection of mycobacteria in clinical specimens. J Clin Microbiol 47(4):1206–1208
20. Baylan O et al (2004) Evaluation of a new automated, rapid, colorimetric culture system using solid medium for laboratory diagnosis of tuberculosis and determination of anti-tuberculosis drug susceptibility. Int J Tuberc Lung Dis 8(6):772–777
21. Neonakis IK et al (2008) Molecular diagnostic tools in mycobacteriology. J Microbiol Methods 75(1):1–11
22. VIncent V, Gutierrez C (2007) Mycobacterium: laboratory characteristics of slowly growing mycobacteria. In: Murray PR (ed) Manual of clinical microbiology. ASM Press, Washington, DC
23. Lefmann M et al (2006) Evaluation of peptide nucleic acid-fluorescence in situ hybridization for identification of clinically relevant mycobacteria in clinical specimens and tissue sections. J Clin Microbiol 44(10):3760–3767
24. Giger O (2007) Mycobacterium tuberculosis and other nonthuberculous mycobacteria. In: Mahon CR, Lehman DC, Manuselis G (eds) Textbook of diagnostic microbiology. Saunders Elsevier, Maryland Heights

25. Tuohy MJ et al (2005) Pyrosequencing as a tool for the identification of common isolates of *Mycobacterium* sp. Diagn Microbiol Infect Dis 51(4):245–250
26. Galor A et al (2007) Rapid species determination of nocardia keratitis using pyrosequencing technology. Am J Ophthalmol 143(1):182–183
27. Chandra NS et al (2001) Cluster of *Mycobacterium chelonae* keratitis cases following laser in-situ keratomileusis. Am J Ophthalmol 132(6):819–830
28. Fulcher SF et al (2002) Delayed-onset mycobacterial keratitis after LASIK. Cornea 21(6): 546–554
29. Chung MS et al (2000) *Mycobacterium chelonae* keratitis after laser in situ keratomileusis successfully treated with medical therapy and flap removal. Am J Ophthalmol 129(3): 382–384
30. de la Cruz J, Pineda R 2nd (2007) LASIK-associated atypical mycobacteria keratitis: a case report and review of the literature. Int Ophthalmol Clin 47(2):73–84
31. Moshirfar M, Meyer JJ, Espandar L (2007) Fourth-generation fluoroquinolone-resistant mycobacterial keratitis after laser in situ keratomileusis. J Cataract Refract Surg 33(11):1978–1981
32. Perez-Balbuena AL (2010) Atypical mycobacterium keratitis associated with penetrating keratoplasty: case report of successful therapy with topical gatifloxacin 0.3%. Cornea 29(4): 468–470
33. Sampaio JL et al (2006) An outbreak of keratitis caused by *Mycobacterium immunogenum*. J Clin Microbiol 44(9):3201–3207
34. Seo KY et al (2002) Non-tuberculous mycobacterial keratitis at the interface after laser in situ keratomileusis. J Refract Surg 18(1):81–85
35. Van Der Beek MT, Bernards AT, Lapid-Gortzak R (2008) *Mycobacterium chelonae* keratitis in a patient with Sjogren's syndrome. Eur J Ophthalmol 18(2):294–296
36. Yamamoto A (2010) *Mycobacterium abscessus* corneal ulcer following sutured clear corneal cataract incision. Jpn J Ophthalmol 54(5):499–500
37. Gelender H et al (2000) Mycobacterium keratitis after laser in situ keratomileusis. J Refract Surg 16(2):191–195
38. Hu FR (1995) Extensive lamellar keratectomy for treatment of nontuberculous mycobacterial keratitis. Am J Ophthalmol 120(1):47–54
39. Srinivasan M, Prajna L, Prajna NV (2005) A cluster of cases of *Mycobacterium chelonei* keratitis following penetrating keratoplasty. Indian J Ophthalmol 53(1):67–68
40. Becero F et al (2002) Keratitis due to *Mycobacterium chelonae* after refractive surgery with LASIK. Enferm Infecc Microbiol Clin 20(1):44–45
41. Griffith DE et al (2007) An official ATS/IDSA statement: diagnosis, treatment, and prevention of nontuberculous mycobacterial diseases. Am J Respir Crit Care Med 175(4):367–416
42. Brown-Elliott BA, Wallace RJ Jr (2002) Clinical and taxonomic status of pathogenic nonpigmented or late-pigmenting rapidly growing mycobacteria. Clin Microbiol Rev 15(4): 716–746
43. Brown-Elliott BA et al (2002) Comparison of in vitro activities of gatifloxacin and ciprofloxacin against four taxa of rapidly growing mycobacteria. Antimicrob Agents Chemother 46(10): 3283–3285
44. Dalovisio JR, Pankey GA (1978) In vitro susceptiiblity of *Mycobacterium fortuitum* and *Mycobacterium chelonei* to amikacin. J Infect Dis 137(3):318–321
45. Fernandez-Roblas R et al (2000) In vitro susceptibilities of rapidly growing mycobacteria to telithromycin (HMR 3647) and seven other antimicrobials. Antimicrob Agents Chemother 44(1):181–182
46. Hu FR et al (1997) The antimicrobial susceptibility of *Mycobacterium chelonae* isolated from corneal ulcer. Curr Eye Res 16(10):1056–1060
47. Reddy AK (2010) In vitro antibiotic susceptibility of rapidly growing nontuberculous mycobacteria isolated from patients with microbial keratitis. Curr Eye Res 35(3):225–229
48. Yang SC et al (2003) High prevalence of antimicrobial resistance in rapidly growing mycobacteria in Taiwan. Antimicrob Agents Chemother 47(6):1958–1962

49. Hofling-Lima AL et al (2005) In vitro activity of fluoroquinolones against *Mycobacterium abscessus* and *Mycobacterium chelonae* causing infectious keratitis after LASIK in Brazil. Cornea 24(6):730–734
50. Hamam RN et al (2006) Recalcitrant post-LASIK *Mycobacterium chelonae* keratitis eradicated after the use of fourth-generation fluoroquinolone. Ophthalmology 113(6):950–954
51. Hu FR, Luh KT (1998) Topical ciprofloxacin for treating nontuberculous mycobacterial keratitis. Ophthalmology 105(2):269–272
52. Bottone EJ, Cho KW (2005) *Mycobacterium chelonae* keratitis: elucidation of diagnosis through evaluation of smears of fluid from patient's contact lens care system. Cornea 24(3): 356–358
53. David DB (1999) *Mycobacterium marinum* keratitis: pigmentation a clue to diagnosis. Eye (Lond) 13(Pt 3a):377–379
54. Matoba AY et al (1993) Combination drug testing of *Mycobacterium chelonae*. Invest Ophthalmol Vis Sci 34(9):2786–2789
55. Hu FR, Wang IJ (1998) Comparison of topical antibiotics for treating *Mycobacterium chelonae* keratitis in a rabbit model. Curr Eye Res 17(5):478–482
56. Wallace RJ Jr et al (2002) Comparison of the in vitro activity of the glycylcycline tigecycline (formerly GAR-936) with those of tetracycline, minocycline, and doxycycline against isolates of nontuberculous mycobacteria. Antimicrob Agents Chemother 46(10):3164–3167
57. Abshire R et al (2004) Topical antibacterial therapy for mycobacterial keratitis: potential for surgical prophylaxis and treatment. Clin Ther 26(2):191–196
58. Gayathri R (2010) Antibiotic susceptibility pattern of rapidly growing mycobacteria. J Postgrad Med 56(2):76–78
59. de la Cruz J, Behlau I, Pineda R (2007) Atypical mycobacteria keratitis after laser in situ keratomileusis unresponsive to fourth-generation fluoroquinolone therapy. J Cataract Refract Surg 33(7):1318–1321
60. Vera-Cabrera L et al (2006) In vitro activities of the novel oxazolidinones DA-7867 and DA-7157 against rapidly and slowly growing mycobacteria. Antimicrob Agents Chemother 50(12):4027–4029
61. Wallace RJ Jr et al (2001) Activities of linezolid against rapidly growing mycobacteria. Antimicrob Agents Chemother 45(3):764–767
62. Rastogi N (2000) In vitro activities of the ketolides telithromycin (HMR 3647) and HMR 3004 compared to those of clarithromycin against slowly growing mycobacteria at pHs 6.8 and 7.4. Antimicrob Agents Chemother 44(10):2848–2852
63. Fernandez-Roblas R et al (2008) In vitro activities of tigecycline and 10 other antimicrobials against nonpigmented rapidly growing mycobacteria. Antimicrob Agents Chemother 52(11): 4184–4186
64. Martin-de-Hijas NZ et al (2008) Usefulness of the Etest for studying tigecycline susceptibility of non-pigmented rapidly growing mycobacteria. Int J Antimicrob Agents 32(4): 366–367
65. Ausina V et al (1986) In vitro activity of clofazimine against rapidly growing nonchromogenic mycobacteria. Antimicrob Agents Chemother 29(5):951–952
66. Ellis BP, Cruickshank JG (1976) Letter: topical clofazimine and atypical mycobacteria. S Afr Med J 50(20):759
67. Shen GH (2010) High efficacy of clofazimine and its synergistic effect with amikacin against rapidly growing mycobacteria. Int J Antimicrob Agents 35(4):400–404
68. Haas W (2010) Bactericidal activity of besifloxacin against staphylococci, *Streptococcus pneumoniae* and *Haemophilus influenzae*. J Antimicrob Chemother 65(7):1441–1447
69. Zhang JZ, Ward KW (2008) Besifloxacin, a novel fluoroquinolone antimicrobial agent, exhibits potent inhibition of pro-inflammatory cytokines in human THP-1 monocytes. J Antimicrob Chemother 61(1):111–116
70. Chung SH et al (2006) *Mycobacterium abscessus* keratitis after LASIK with IntraLase femtosecond laser. Ophthalmologica 220(4):277–280

71. Lois N, Perez del Molino ML (1995) *Mycobacterium chelonae* keratitis: resolution after debridement and presoaked collagen shields. Cornea 14(5):536–539
72. Susiyanti M, Mehta JS, Tan DT (2007) Bilateral deep anterior lamellar keratoplasty for the management of bilateral post-LASIK mycobacterial keratitis. J Cataract Refract Surg 33(9):1641–1643
73. Makdoumi K, Mortensen J, Crafoord S (2010) Infectious keratitis treated with corneal cross-linking. Cornea 29(12):1353–1358
74. Micelli Ferrari T (2009) *Escherichia coli* keratitis treated with ultraviolet A/riboflavin corneal cross-linking: a case report. Eur J Ophthalmol 19(2):295–297
75. Pollhammer M, Cursiefen C (2009) Bacterial keratitis early after corneal crosslinking with riboflavin and ultraviolet-A. J Cataract Refract Surg 35(3):588–589
76. Sharma N (2010) Pseudomonas keratitis after collagen crosslinking for keratoconus: case report and review of literature. J Cataract Refract Surg 36(3):517–520

New Developments in Antibacterial Chemotherapy for Bacterial Keratitis

2

H. Sueke, J. Shankar, T.J. Neal, M. Horsburgh, R. Gilbert, and Stephen B. Kaye

Core Messages

- The treatment of bacterial keratitis depends on identifying the causative agent and selecting an appropriate antimicrobial.
- The initial antimicrobial that is prescribed should be selected based on
  (i) The most likely causative bacterium, from contemporaneous clinical and laboratory data (bacterial spectrum and antimicrobial studies)
  (ii) Knowledge of the pharmacokinetics and pharmacodynamics of the agent
- Treatment is then modified based on
  (i) Actual bacterial species identified
  (ii) Antimicrobial susceptibility assays
  (iii) Clinical response
- Antimicrobial combination therapy should be based on those combinations
  (i) Which are likely to produce a synergistic response
  (ii) For which the suspected or isolated bacteria are likely to be susceptible
- Antimicrobial combinations which increase the antimicrobial spectrum but which are likely to be antagonistic or inhibitory should not be used.

H. Sueke (✉) • J. Shankar • R. Gilbert • S.B. Kaye
St. Paul's Eye Unit, Royal Liverpool University Hospital,
8Z Link, Prescot Street, Liverpool L7 8XP, UK
e-mail: hsueke@liverpool.ac.uk; jayendra.shankar@liv.ac.uk; s.b.kaye@liverpool.ac.uk

T.J. Neal
Department of Microbiology, Royal Liverpool University Hospital,
7th floor, Duncan Building, Daulby street, Liverpool L69 3GA, UK
e-mail: t.j.neal@lic.ac.uk

M. Horsburgh
Institute of Integrative Biology, University of Liverpool, Crown street,
Liverpool L69 7ZB, UK
e-mail: m.j.horsburgh@liv.ac.uk

T. Reinhard, F. Larkin (eds.), *Corneal Disease*,
DOI 10.1007/978-3-642-28747-3_2, © Springer-Verlag Berlin Heidelberg 2013

- Host and bacterial factors and their interaction must also be considered as they both play a crucial role in determining clinical outcome and the risk of recurrent disease.
  (i) Specific host risk factors should be identified such as ocular surface disease.
  (ii) Bacterial isolates should be kept and investigated for known virulence factors.
- The relevant contribution or interaction of host and bacterial factors to the clinical outcome may be dependent on the individual patient. Future treatment of recurrent disease needs to be tailored according to the relevant contribution of host and bacterial factors in the individual patient. An example might be recurrent *Staphylococcus aureus* corneal ulceration in a patient with chronic meibomian gland disease with nasal colonisation by PVL-producing *Staphylococcus aureus*.
- Novel antimicrobials under evaluation include besifloxacin, meropenem, tigecycline and linezolid

Introduction

The ideal treatment of bacterial keratitis depends on identifying the causative agent and selecting an appropriate antimicrobial. The initial antimicrobial that is prescribed, however, is selected based on the most likely causative bacteria from contemporaneous clinical and laboratory data (bacterial spectrum and antimicrobial studies) and knowledge of the pharmacokinetics and pharmacodynamics of the agent. Treatment is then modified based on the actual bacterium identified and its antimicrobial susceptibility assays, and clinical response. In addition, host and non-antimicrobial virulence factors must also be considered as they both play a crucial role in determining clinical outcome and the risk of recurrent disease.

Epidemiology

The epidemiological patterns of bacterial keratitis vary with patient population, health of the cornea, geographic location and climate. Bacteria are responsible for a larger proportion of corneal ulceration in temperate climates such as the United Kingdom and northern United States than in tropical regions such as south India, where fungal infection predominates [1]. There are approximately 6,000 cases of bacterial keratitis per year in the UK (c.150 per year for a city the size of Liverpool or Manchester).

Visual Morbidity

Bacterial keratitis leads to severe inflammation, thinning, distortion, vascularisation and scarring of the cornea. The severity of the infection correlates positively with increased scarring and corresponding loss of vision. Many cases require hospitalisation with prolonged treatment periods. Bacterial keratitis accounts for approximately 8% of corneal transplants undertaken in the UK [Ocular Tissue Advisory Group to NHS BT UK]. Patients with an abnormal ocular surface from neurotrophic keratopathy, herpes simplex keratitis, Sjogrens syndrome and contact lens wearers, may have different responses to treatment despite having the same bacteria isolated from their corneal ulcer.

Documentation

Attention to clinical detail is helpful in recognising clues to the aetiological agent (characteristics of the corneal ulcer), host factors (presence of ocular surface disease) and for monitoring the clinical response. Precise and accurate documentation and recording of the condition is therefore important, and photography or detailed drawings (Fig. 2.1 [2]) are needed.

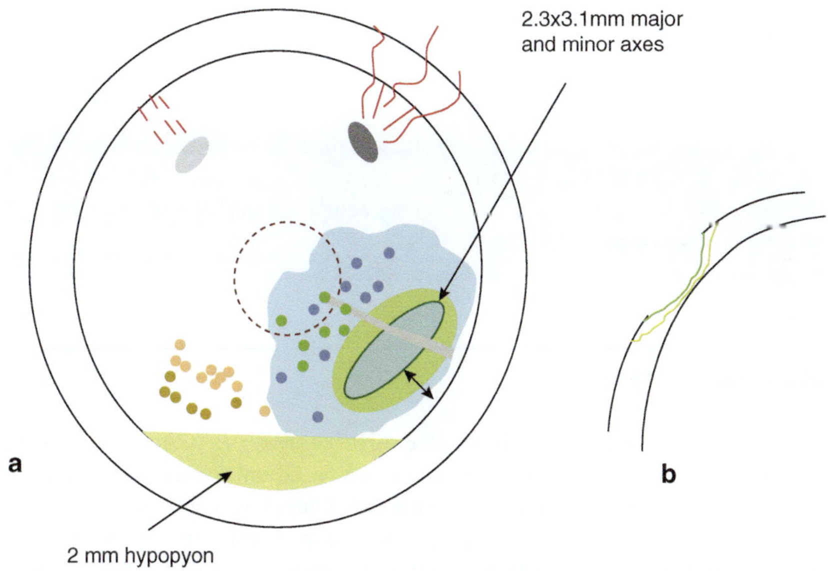

Fig. 2.1 Drawing of corneal ulcer (adapted from Waring et al. [2]) (**a**) anterior posterior view, (**b**) cross section through ulcer. *Black continues circle*, corneal limbus; *outer dashed line*, contact lens. *Blue shade*, stromal oedema; *blue dots*, epithelial oedema. *Green dots*, punctate keratopathy; *green line*, epithelial defect. *Red straight hashed lines*, ghost vessels; *straight lines*, deep stromal vessels; *wavy lines*, superficial vessels. *Grey oval shapes*: light grey, old scar; dark grey recent scar. *Orange and brown dots*: new and old keratitic precipitates. *Yellow shade*: hypopyon, corneal infiltrates and abscess formation. *Brown hashed circle*: pupil

Summary for the Clinician

- Bacterial keratitis almost always results in a corneal scar
- Good accurate documentation is required in follow up of corneal ulcers

Causative Factors

Predisposing factors that facilitate successful bacterial colonisation and invasion of the cornea include trauma, contact lens wear, ocular surface disease [3, 4] and corneal surface abnormalities [5]. These are all significant risk factors and often are associated with recurrent disease [6]. Although the majority of patients have one or more risk factors, contact lens use is seen as the major risk factor in most studies [5, 6]. Lam et al. [7] reported that the incidence of bacterial keratitis was sixfold higher in contact lens wearers than in the general population and an increased incidence of *Pseudomonas aeruginosa* (*P. aeruginosa*) infections coincided with the increased popularity of contact lens wear. Among contact lens users, extended-wear contact lens wearers are at an increased risk of bacterial infection relative to daily disposable lens wearers [3]. Contact lens wear and correspondingly, contact lens-related keratitis is rarer in developing countries [4].

Summary for the Clinician

- In treating bacterial keratitis, host factors must be considered; they may be indicators for recurrent disease.
- Risk factors include contact lens use, ocular surface disease, trauma and Sjogrens Syndrome.

Causative Bacteria

Of the bacteria associated with an ulcerative keratitis, *P. aeruginosa*, a Gram-negative bacillus, and *Staphylococcus aureus*, a Gram-positive coccus, are the most common bacterial pathogens. Although coagulase-negative staphylococci (CNS) account for a significant proportion of bacteria that are isolated from patients with bacterial keratitis, they are found in the conjunctival flora [8, 9] and their primary role in the disease is unclear. For example, a recent study has shown a positive correlation between clinical outcome and in vitro susceptibility for *S. aureus* and *P. aeruginosa*, but not for CNS [10]. Although *Streptococci* spp. are isolated less commonly, *Strep. pneumoniae* is often associated with a poor outcome and accounts for the greatest percentage of cases where eyes are lost [10]. Prompt intervention is crucial if a *Strep. pneumoniae*-related keratitis is suspected.

Table 2.1 Percentage of different bacterial species from patients with bacterial keratitis: comparable studies

Organism	Sueke [11] (UK) $n=772$	Tuft [12] (UK) $n=1,312$	Bourcier [5] (France) $n=208$	Bharati [13] (India) $n=1,109$
Gram-positive bacteria				
Coagulase-negative staphylococci	26.9	N/A	48.1	17.4
Methicillin sensitive	21.7	N/A	N/A	N/A
Methicillin resistant	5.2	N/A	N/A	N/A
Staphylococcus aureus	13.6	33.4	7.7	3.9
Methicillin sensitive	12.4	N/A	N/A	N/A
Methicillin resistant	1.2	N/A	N/A	N/A
Streptococcus	12.6	19.0	9.2	42.4
Strep. pneumoniae	3.4	N/A	3.4	37.5
Other alpha-haemolytic	7.8	N/A	5.8	4.4
Beta-haemolytic[a]	1.4	N/A	N/A	0.5
Other Gram-positive[b]	4.4	3.5	17.8	6.3
Gram-positives subtotal	57.4	55.9	82.8	70.1
Gram-negative bacteria				
Pseudomonas aeruginosa	20.9	24.8	10.1	18.0
Enterobacteriaceae	13.4	8.5	6.3	1.1
Serratia spp.	4.4	3.0	5.3	0.2
Klebsiella spp.	2.1	0.4	N/A	0.4
Citrobacter spp.	1.6	0.4	N/A	2.6
Proteus spp.	1.6	0.7	1.0	N/A
E. coli	1.2	0.6	N/A	N/A
Enterobacter spp.	1.0	2.1	N/A	0.8
Morganella morganii	0.1	N/A	N/A	0.5
Pantoea spp.	0.1	N/A	N/A	N/A
Other	1.2	1.3	N/A	29.9
Moraxella spp.	2.6	5.9	0.5	N/A
Haemophilus spp.	1.4	2.2	N/A	N/A
Other Gram-negatives[c]	4.2	2.8	N/A	N/A
Gram-negatives subtotal	42.5	44.2	16.9	20.9

[a]Lancefield Group A (0.3%), Group B (0.1%), Group C (0.3%), Group G (0.8%)
[b]*Corynebacterium* spp. (2.6%), *Bacillus* spp. (1.7%), *Enterococcus* spp. (0.9%), *Listeria* spp. (0.1%)
[c]*Acinetobacter* spp. (1.2%), *Stenotrophomonas maltophilia* (1.2%), *Neisseria* spp. (0.3%), *Pasturella* spp. (0.3%), *Aeromonas* spp. (0.1%), *Eikenella* spp. (0.1%), *Agrobacterium* spp. (0.1%), *Alcaligines* spp. (0.1%), *Methylbacterium* spp. (0.1%)

Table 2.1 illustrates the wide variability in the proportions of bacteria causing keratitis between four similar studies set in different geographical locations. For example, the proportion of Gram-positive isolates varies between 56% and 83% and the proportion of Gram-negative isolates varies between 17% and 44%. Differences may reflect climate of the country or prevalence of risk factors such as contact lens use, trauma or co-existent ocular disease.

Summary for the Clinician

- Causative bacteria and host factors can vary significantly between geographical locations.
- *Streptococcus pneumoniae* is associated with the worst outcomes and requires prompt treatment.

Investigation of Keratitis

There are various approaches to the microbiological investigation of patients with suspected keratitis. Traditional methods include the use of multiple corneal scrapes with direct inoculation onto different enrichment media. Collecting multiple scrapes, particularly from the eye of an uncooperative patient, is not always easy. Growing a minute sample in culture on an agar plate is technically difficult: the inoculum might be deposited beneath the surface of the agar, a full range of fresh culture media may not be always available and the non-laboratory setting poses an increased risk of extraneous contamination of culture plates. These problems explain the reluctance of some ophthalmologists to perform a corneal scrape to reach a microbiological diagnosis. For example, McDonnell et al. [14] found that 49% of ophthalmologists treated corneal ulcers empirically without attempting to identify the causative organism. Kaye et al. [15] reported that collecting two corneal scrapes, one for a smear and the other placed in an enrichment transport medium (such as brain heart infusion broth), resulted in detection rates similar to those of direct plating with no significant loss of organisms.

The role of polymerase chain reaction (PCR) techniques has recently been evaluated to diagnose bacterial keratitis [16, 17]. PCR has the advantage of being a quicker and more sensitive technique than traditional culture methods; however, its high sensitivity may result in false-positive results. Although further larger studies comparing the two techniques are necessary to evaluate its place in the diagnosis of bacterial keratitis, it would seem reasonable to include PCR as part of the patient's investigation.

Laboratory Diagnosis: Susceptibility Testing

Topical antimicrobials form the mainstay of treatment of bacterial keratitis. Despite their widespread usage, clinical decision making has rested upon susceptibility data derived from and for systemic infections. The relationship between bacterial susceptibility to antimicrobials and clinical outcome has only recently been demonstrated [10]. Although there are significant associations between the minimum inhibitory concentration of the prescribed antimicrobial and the clinical outcome, the parameters of the association may be dependent on the particular bacterial species and antimicrobial.

Susceptibility and Resistance of Bacterial Isolates

The basic laboratory measurement of the activity of an antimicrobial is the MIC, which is defined as the lowest antimicrobial concentration that will inhibit overnight growth of bacteria. The MIC is used to determine the susceptibility and resistance of an antimicrobial, by comparing it to a set of standard MICs based on the safe achievable concentrations of antimicrobial in the serum. Standards are set by the Clinical and Laboratory Standards Institute in the United States and British Society for Antimicrobial Chemotherapy (BSAC) in the UK. Interpreting resistance and susceptibility needs to be done with caution, as currently there are no standards for topical ocular therapy that relate to the concentrations of antimicrobial in ocular tissue. For example, Sueke et al. [11] found the range of MICs for ciprofloxacin against 140 *P. aeruginosa* isolates to be 0.016 to 6.0 mg/L. Using the breakpoint figure of 1.0 mg/L from BSAC, which was calculated from systemic data, 98% of isolates were susceptible to ciprofloxacin. These figures can be expressed graphically in comparison to the other three fluoroquinolones tested (Fig. 2.2). The MIC_{90} is a descriptive statistic estimating the antimicrobial concentration which will inhibit the growth of 90% of isolates and the MIC_{50} is the concentration which inhibits 50% of isolates. Figure 2.3 illustrates the MICs of ciprofloxacin against 126 *S. aureus* isolates. Antimicrobial concentrations that are achieved in the cornea and aqueous are indicated on the graph.

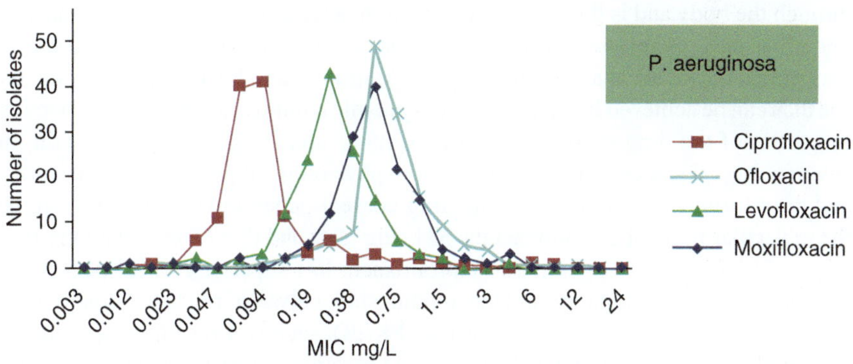

Fig. 2.2 Minimum inhibitory concentrations (mg/L) of four fluoroquinolones against 160 *P. aeruginosa* isolates collected from patients in the United Kingdom with bacterial keratitis [11]

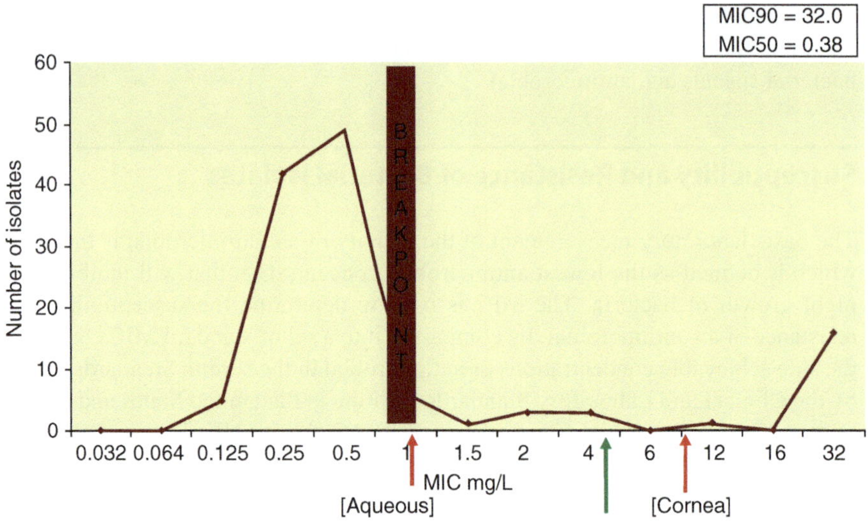

Fig. 2.3 Minimum inhibitory concentrations (mg/L) of ciprofloxacin against 126 *S. aureus* isolates taken from the United Kingdom from patients with bacterial keratitis [11]. Also annotated on the graph are concentrations of ciprofloxacin in the aqueous and cornea (*red arrow*, chemical concentration; *green arrow*, bioassay concentration) [18]

Treatment: Antimicrobials

The efficacy of an antimicrobial in the cornea is dependent on the relationship between its pharmacodynamic and pharmacokinetic properties.

Pharmacodynamics, the effect of the drug on the bacteria, is measured by determining its MIC, as defined above. Pharmacokinetics is the ability of the drug to pass through the body and is therefore also crucial in determining the efficacy of an antimicrobial in treating bacterial keratitis. Topical application of an antimicrobial to the cornea may achieve a very different concentration and bioavailability in the tissue than can be achieved in the serum after systemic administration. Physicochemical properties of the drug such as lipophilicity, molecular weight, pH, and stability in solution may play a critical part. In addition, physiological properties of the cornea and drug formulation may determine drug corneal penetration [19]. For example, the molecular mass of ciprofloxacin is 331 (Fig. 2.4) and that of teicoplanin is 1907 (Fig. 2.5) which may explain why ciprofloxacin has superior corneal penetration than teicoplanin [18]. Studying the relationship between pharmacokinetics and pharmacodynamics (otherwise known as PK/PD analysis) results in a complete overall understanding of how a drug works in practice. This has recently been studied in bacterial keratitis for ciprofloxacin and teicoplanin. Kaye et al. [10] compared the differences between the predicted (tissue concentration based upon chemical measurement) and actual activity of an antimicrobial based upon a bioassay (measurement of antimicrobial activity in the tissue). They found a significant difference

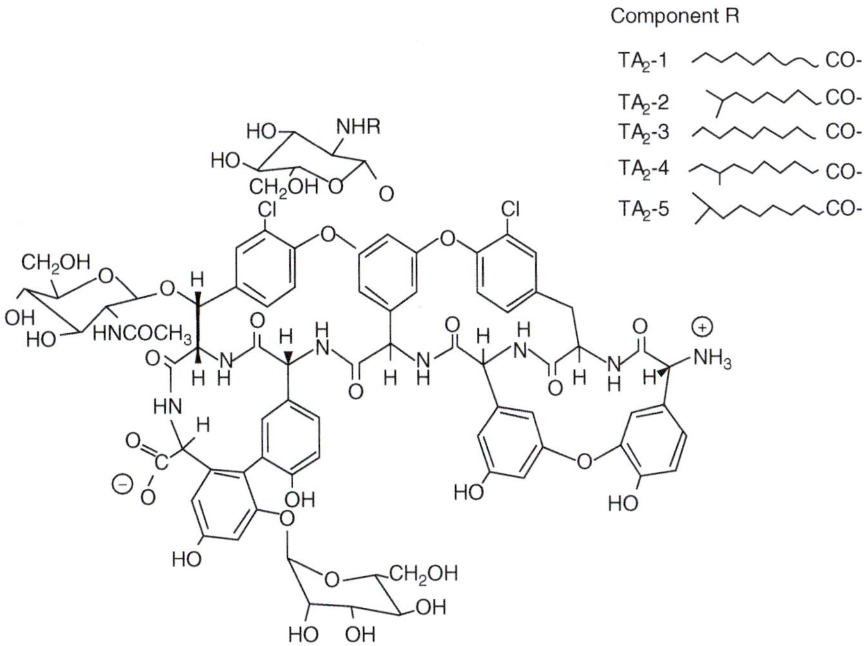

Fig. 2.4 Molecular structure of teicoplanin: molecular mass 1,907

Fig. 2.5 Molecular structure of ciprofloxacin: molecular mass 331

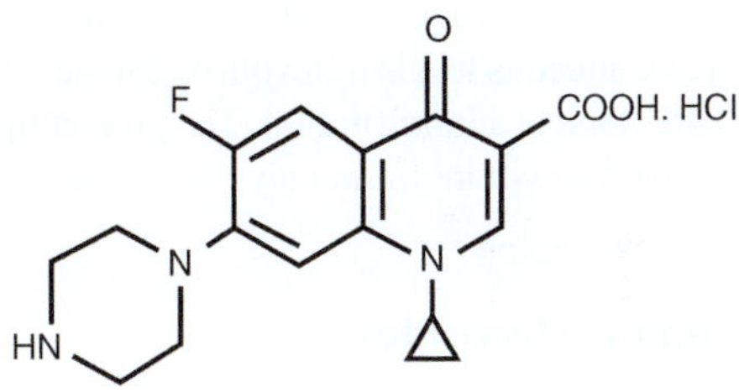

between the chemical concentration and biological activity of ciprofloxacin following topical administration to the cornea.

Current Antimicrobials in Use

The ophthalmologist has a number of potential antimicrobials at their disposal to treat bacterial keratitis. When choosing an antimicrobial prior to the results of bacterial culture and sensitivity, the choice of one drug over another may be determined by a variety of factors, for example local bacterial epidemiology, drug cost, and drug toxicity.

The Fluoroquinolones

The development of an old class of antimicrobials, the fluoroquinolones, in the 1990s, provided for the first time a class of drugs with broad Gram-positive and Gram-negative activity and little corneal toxicity [20]. Fluoroquinolones work by inhibiting DNA gyrase (also known as Topoisomerase II) and topoisomerase IV, enzymes necessary in bacterial DNA synthesis. Second-generation fluoroquinolones, ciprofloxacin (see Fig. 2.4) and ofloxacin, are widely used in treating bacterial keratitis. They offer a great potency against Gram-negative bacilli (including *P. aeruginosa)*, moderate activity against *S. aureus* and little activity against streptococci and the pneumococci. Despite the success of the first- and second-generation fluoroquinolones, there has been a trend (based on systemic breakpoints) towards an increase in resistance of both *S. aureus* [21] and *P. aeruginosa* [22].

Further molecular modifications of the fluoroquinolones in 2000s lead to the development of the third-generation levofloxacin, and the fourth-generation moxifloxacin and gatifloxacin. These agents have greater potency against Gram-positive bacteria, in particular the Streptococci. The later-generation fluoroquinolones unfortunately have not been a treatment panacea because of the emergence of resistance (albeit based on systemic breakpoint data) [23, 24]. Park et al. [25] showed a rate of 2% resistance (based again on systemic breakpoint data) to moxifloxacin and 5% to gatifloxacin in isolates of normal bacterial ocular flora. Sueke et al. [11] showed a rate of 2% resistance using systemic breakpoint data to moxifloxacin and 16% to ciprofloxacin in *S. aureus* isolates from patients with bacterial keratitis. A number of pharmacokinetic studies have shown moxifloxacin to have superior corneal penetration compared to the other fluoroquinolones [26–28]. For example, in a rabbit endophthalmitis model [28], aqueous levels of levofloxacin were 9.4 mg/L, and moxifloxacin was 43.3 mg/L after topical administration. The greater lipophilicity of moxifloxacin compared to the other fluoroquinolones may explain this phenomenon.

Aminoglycosides

Aminoglycosides such as gentamicin and tobramicin are often used in treating bacterial keratitis. They have a broad range of bactericidal activity against many bacterial species, particularly Gram-negative rods. They have an affinity to bacterial 30 S and 50 S ribosomal subunits producing a non-functional 70 S initiation complex resulting in an inhibition of protein synthesis. They are sometimes given in combination with predominantly Gram-positive antimicrobials. Their use is limited by their associated corneal toxicity [29].

Sueke et al. [11] showed gentamicin to have 4% resistance using systemic breakpoints against *S. aureus* and *P. aeruginosa*, whereas amikacin had no resistance to *S. aureus* and 4% to *P. aeruginosa*. Gentamicin has, however, been shown to have poor corneal penetration which may be due to the hydrophobic nature of the compound. Baum et al. [30] showed that the concentration of gentamicin in the aqueous at 1 hour is only 1 mg/L, which is lower than the suggested MIC using systemic breakpoints.

Cephalosporins

Cephalosporins have a broad spectrum of activity, including effective action against *Haemophilus* species. They contain a β-lactam ring similar to penicillin but have the advantage of being resistant to the penicillinases. They inhibit bacterial cell wall synthesis and are well tolerated topically. The first-generation cephalosporins include cephazolin, second-generation cefuroxime and third-generation ceftazidime. Cefuroxime has often been used in combination with an aminoglycoside for the empirical treatment of suspected bacterial keratitis. Cefuroxime and ceftazidime had high MICs against *S. aureus* and *P. aeruginosa* suggesting a significant degree of antimicrobial resistance; however, systemic breakpoints were not available to formally assess this. Jenkins et al. [31] found that following topical administration to cataract surgery patients, aqueous concentrations of cefuroxime were only significant when applied once the corneal wound had been fashioned. This suggests poor corneal penetration of cefuroxime which may be explained as the cephalosporins are hydrophobic [31].

Other Antimicrobials Used

Glycopeptides such as teicoplanin and vancomycin have activity against Gram-positive bacteria, including methicillin and penicillin-resistant staphylococci. They inhibit the biosynthesis of peptidoglycan polymers during the second stage of bacterial cell wall formation, at a different site of action from that of the β-lactam antimicrobials. They also have an excellent activity against a variety of Gram-positive bacilli, but not Gram-negative bacteria which are inherently resistant. The glycopeptides are, however, large molecules and in the intact corneal epithelium show a reduced corneal penetration, as mentioned previously [18].

Summary for the Clinician

- The fluoroquinolones provide good activity against Gram-negative and most Gram-positive bacteria causing an ulcerative keratitis, although resistance of the latter is emerging.
- Additional specific Gram-positive coverage is offered by teicoplanin or vancomycin.

Development of Existing and New Classes of Drugs

Besifloxacin

Besifloxacin is a novel fluoroquinolone for topical ophthalmic use, recently approved by the US Food and Drug Administration (USFDA) for the treatment of bacterial conjunctivitis [32]. Besifloxacin appears to have a broad spectrum of activity against aerobic and anaerobic bacteria, possibly due to its cyclopropyl group and chloride substituent at C-8 improving its activity against DNA gyrase and topoisomerase IV enzymes. Besifloxacin has been shown to be active against both Gram-positive (S. *aureus*, *Strep. pneumoniae*, *Corynebacterium* and *Propionibacterium acnes*) and Gram-negative organisms (*H. influenzae*, *Moraxella*, *Escherichia coli*, *Neisseria gonorrhoeae* and *P. aeruginosa*). Recent studies have found besifloxacin to have good pharmacokinetic parameters in vitro [33] as well as excellent efficacy in animal models of keratitis, compared to fourth-generation fluoroquinolones [34, 35].

Tigecycline

Tigecycline [36] is a glycylcycline with activity against most aerobic and anaerobic Gram-positive and -negative bacteria but with limited activity against *P. aeruginosa*. Glycylcyclines are bacteriostatic agents that inhibit protein synthesis in bacteria by reversibly binding to the 30 S ribosomal subunit. Sueke et al. [27] showed tigecycline to have no resistance to any Gram-positive isolates using systemic breakpoints, but complete resistance to *P. aeruginosa*. Corneal pharmacokinetics of tigecycline, however, have not yet been determined.

Linezolid

Linezolid [37], the first of a new class, the oxazolidinones, is a synthetic compound with activity against all the major Gram-positive groups of bacteria, but no activity against Gram-negative bacteria. Linezolid works by inhibiting bacterial ribosomal protein synthesis by binding to a site on the 50 S ribosomal subunit, thus preventing the formation of a 70 S initiation complex. Pharmacokinetic studies using animal models of keratitis have showed good corneal penetration and no recorded toxicity with linezolid [38, 39]. Sueke et al. [11] showed linezolid to have no resistance against Gram-positive isolates including methicillin-resistant *S. aureus*.

Meropenem

Meropenem [40] is a broad-spectrum carbapenem that is currently FDA approved to treat skin infections, intraabdominal infections and bacterial meningitis. Like other carbapenems, it is a β-lactam antimicrobial, working through bacterial cell wall inhibition. It has activity against Gram-positive and -negative pathogens, including extended-spectrum lactamases (ESBL) and AmpC-producing Enterobacteriaceae. Sueke et al. [11] showed meropenem to have wide coverage against both Gram-positive and Gram-negative microorganisms, where only one of the 772 isolates tested (*P. aeruginosa*) was resistant using systemic breakpoints. Corneal pharmacokinetics of meropenem are not yet known; however, intravitreal meropenem in a rabbit model of endophthalmitis [41] did not show any evidence of toxicity.

Similarly, intravenous meropenem prior to cataract surgery showed penetration of the drug into the anterior chamber with no notable side effects [42].

Developing Ophthalmic Breakpoints: Relation Between MIC and Clinical Outcome

There is good evidence demonstrating the relationship between the MIC of topically applied antimicrobials and clinical outcome in bacterial keratitis [10]. This relationship is particularly well established for pathogenic bacteria such as *P. aeruginosa* and *S. aureus*. Figure 2.6 summarises the relationship for the patients in a study by Kaye et al. [10] between a measure of clinical outcome (healing time to ulcer size: HT/UA) and the lowest MIC of the particular antimicrobial agent used. The general linear multivariate model revealed a weak but significant association between the MIC of the antimicrobial prescribed and clinical outcome defined by the ratio of healing time to ulcer size. The importance of the bacterial type and antimicrobial used for treatment is indicated by the significant associations between the fluoroquinolone MIC and clinical outcome for *Pseudomonas* spp., *S. aureus* and *Enterobacteriaceae* but not for *Streptococcus* spp. or CNS. The MIC is therefore an important measure for evaluating the potential effectiveness of topically applied antimicrobials in the treatment of bacterial keratitis.

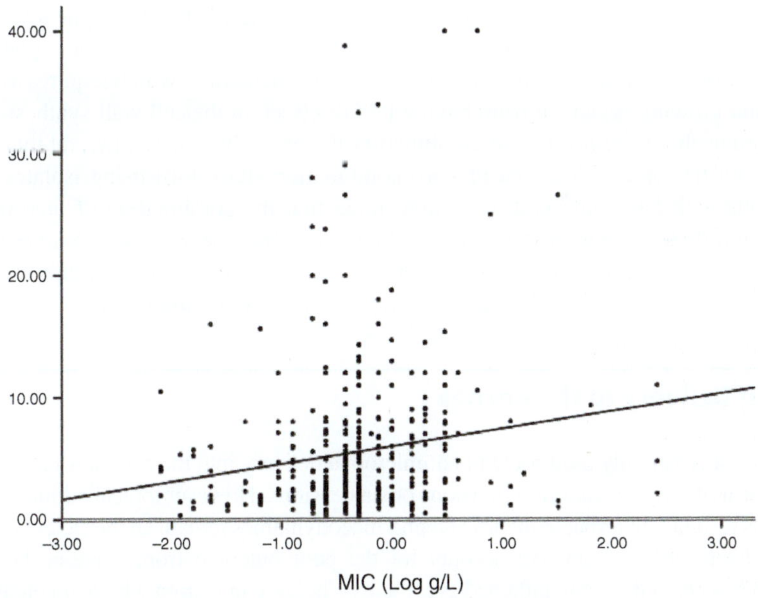

Fig. 2.6 Clinical outcome and MIC: antimicrobial used and all bacterial isolates. Healing time to ulcer area (HT/UA) (days per mm²), logarithm (Log) of Minimum inhibitory concentration (MIC mg/L). Hypothetical susceptible and resistant outcomes (HT/UA of 3.5 and 7 days/mm²) corresponds to an MIC of 0.1 and 10 mg/L [10]

Summary for the Clinician

- The minimum inhibitory concentration (MIC) is defined as the lowest antimicrobial concentration that will inhibit overnight growth of bacteria.
- A relationship has now been determined between MIC and clinical outcome for *S. aureus* and *P. aeruginosa*.

Combination Therapy

As opposed to single therapy, an antimicrobial combination offers a broader spectrum of activity and may reduce selective pressures. This may be of particular importance for the fluoroquinolones, as increasing resistance has been reported in *S. aureus* and *P. aeruginosa* isolates from cases of bacterial keratitis [9, 21–24]. An often overlooked reason for combination therapy, however, is not for providing a broader spectrum but for an increased antimicrobial effect. In particular, combination therapy may result in synergy as occurs, for example, with the combination of penicillin and gentamicin when used in the treatment of enterococcal endocarditis [43, 44]. This synergistic effect can be explained by the increased ease of gentamicin passage into the bacterial cell, due to cell wall disruption caused by the action of penicillin. Conversely, combinations of antimicrobials may be antagonistic, as occurs with the combination of chloramphenicol and penicillin in the treatment of pneumococcal meningitis [45]. The presumed reason for this antagonism is that chloramphenicol, a bacteriostatic agent, by reducing growth prevents penicillin, which requires a dividing and growing organism from having its full effect on the cell wall synthesis. It is important therefore not to use combination therapy which may have inhibitory or antagonistic effects. A recent in vitro combination study [46] using isolates from patients with bacterial keratitis demonstrated that the combination of meropenem and ciprofloxacin was predominantly additive or synergistic for both *S. aureus* and *P. aeruginosa*. Furthermore, teicoplanin combined with meropenem, ciprofloxacin or moxifloxacin was also additive or synergistic against *S. aureus*.

Drug Delivery to the Cornea

The most commonly used route of antimicrobial delivery into the cornea is topically, in the form of drops, solutions, emulsions or suspensions. However topical administration and its resultant pharmacokinetics and pharmacodynamics remain an inefficient method of delivery and may in part account for the poor outcome from bacterial keratitis. Furthermore, in the acute inflamed eye, there is increase in tearing which, together with the associated pain, makes instillation of a topical antimicrobial difficult. Hospitalisation is often needed to deliver the antimicrobials at frequent intervals (15 min) through consecutive nights. It is clear therefore that drug delivery systems need to be rethought.

Novel Methods of Drug Delivery to the Cornea

Alternative methods of delivery of antimicrobials to treat keratitis are currently being studied [47, 48]. Various drug delivery devices have been evaluated for the treatment of keratitis. They broadly fall into two categories: matrix and reservoir based. Matrix-based implants distribute the drug throughout a degradable polymer matrix, for example, Lacrisert® [49]. In a reservoir implant, the drug is stored within a reservoir made of a non-degradable substance such as collagen shields. Drug penetration into the cornea can be also enhanced by altering its physicochemical properties with the addition of particulates such as nano-particles and other penetration enhancers, as well as using the prodrug and mucoadhesive dosage forms.

Summary for the Clinician

- Resistance to commonly used antimicrobials in keratitis has prompted the development of novel strategies in treating bacterial keratitis.
- Novel antimicrobials such as besifloxacin, tigecycline, meropenem and linezolid are currently under consideration.
- Additional improvements to clinical outcome may arise through utilising synergistic combinations of antimicrobials, as well as using novel corneal drug delivery systems.

Conclusion

It is clear that although there is a significant relationship between the MIC of the prescribed topical antimicrobial and clinical outcome, this relationship is relatively small; c.14%. Other bacterial and host factors play a role in the progression of infection. This is underlined by the finding that although the majority of bacterial isolates from keratitis based upon systemic breakpoint data were reported to be susceptible to prescribed antimicrobials, the actual outcome was far worse than expected. It is clear therefore that although ophthalmic susceptibility data to topical antimicrobials gives a better indication of outcome, the main determinants of outcome relate to factors such as the host–bacterial interaction. This is particularly evident for infections caused by *S. aureus* which accounts for up to 31% of cases of keratitis with the majority of ocular surface infections occurring in patients living in the community in the United Kingdom. This nevertheless presents an opportunity to develop treatments aimed at interfering with the action of the bacteria on its host target. These treatments could also be delivered in novel ways, reducing the dependency of instilling intensive topical antimicrobials.

References

1. Bharathi MJ et al (2007) Microbial keratitis in South India: influence of risk factors, climate, and geographical variation. Ophthalmic Epidemiol 14(2):61–69
2. Waring GO, Laibson PR (1977) A systematic method of drawing corneal pathologic conditions. Arch Ophthalmol 95(9):1540–1542
3. Liesegang TJ (1997) Contact lens-related microbial keratitis: part I: epidemiology. Cornea 16(2):125–131
4. Sharma S et al (2003) Trends in contact lens-associated microbial keratitis in Southern India. Ophthalmology 110(1):138–143
5. Bourcier T et al (2003) Bacterial keratitis: predisposing factors, clinical and microbiological review of 300 cases. Br J Ophthalmol 87(7):834–838
6. Schaefer F et al (2001) Bacterial keratitis: a prospective clinical and microbiological study. Br J Ophthalmol 85(7):842–847
7. Lam DS et al (2002) Incidence and risk factors for microbial keratitis in Hong Kong: comparison with Europe and North America. Eye (Lond) 16(5):608–618
8. Fahmy JA, Moller S, Bentzon MW (1974) Bacterial flora of the normal conjunctiva. I. Topographical distribution. Acta Ophthalmol (Copenh) 52(6):786–800
9. Fukuda M et al (2002) Methicillin-resistant *Staphylococcus aureus* and methicillin-resistant coagulase-negative *Staphylococcus* ocular surface infection efficacy of chloramphenicol eye drops. Cornea 21(7 Suppl):S86–S89
10. Kaye S et al (2010) Bacterial susceptibility to topical antimicrobials and clinical outcome in bacterial keratitis. Invest Ophthalmol Vis Sci 51(1):362–368
11. Sueke H et al (2010) Minimum inhibitory concentrations of standard and novel antimicrobials for isolates from bacterial keratitis. Invest Ophthalmol Vis Sci 51(5):2519–2524
12. Tuft SJ, Matheson M (2000) In vitro antibiotic resistance in bacterial keratitis in London. Br J Ophthalmol 84(7):687–691
13. Bharathi MJ et al (2003) Epidemiology of bacterial keratitis in a referral centre in south India. Indian J Med Microbiol 21(4):239–245
14. McDonnell PJ (1996) Empirical or culture-guided therapy for microbial keratitis? A plea for data. Arch Ophthalmol 114(1):84–87
15. Kaye SB et al (2003) Simplifying collection of corneal specimens in cases of suspected bacterial keratitis. J Clin Microbiol 41(7):3192–3197
16. Itahashi M et al (2010) Detection and quantification of pathogenic bacteria and fungi using real-time polymerase chain reaction by cycling probe in patients with corneal ulcer. Arch Ophthalmol 128(5):535–540
17. Subrayan V et al (2010) Assessment of polymerase chain reaction in the detection of *Pseudomonas aeruginosa* in contact lens-induced severe infectious keratitis. Eye Contact Lens 36(4):201–203
18. Kaye SB et al (2009) Concentration and bioavailability of ciprofloxacin and teicoplanin in the cornea. Invest Ophthalmol Vis Sci 50(7):3176–3184
19. Urtti A (2006) Challenges and obstacles of ocular pharmacokinetics and drug delivery. Adv Drug Deliv Rev 58(11):1131–1135
20. Baum J, Barza M (2000) The evolution of antibiotic therapy for bacterial conjunctivitis and keratitis: 1970–2000. Cornea 19(5):659–672
21. Goldstein MH, Kowalski RP, Gordon YJ (1999) Emerging fluoroquinolone resistance in bacterial keratitis: a 5-year review. Ophthalmology 106(7):1313–1318
22. Garg P, Sharma S, Rao GN (1999) Ciprofloxacin-resistant *Pseudomonas* keratitis. Ophthalmology 106(7):1319–1323
23. Moshirfar M et al (2006) Fourth-generation fluoroquinolone-resistant bacterial keratitis after refractive surgery. J Cataract Refract Surg 32(3):515–518
24. Jhanji V et al (2007) Fourth-generation fluoroquinolone-resistant bacterial keratitis. J Cataract Refract Surg 33(8):1488–1489
25. Park SH et al (2009) The resistance patterns of normal ocular bacterial flora to 4 fluoroquinolone antibiotics. Cornea 28(1):68–72

26. Kim DH, Stark WJ, O'Brien TP (2005) Ocular penetration of moxifloxacin 0.5% and gatifloxacin 0.3% ophthalmic solutions into the aqueous humor following topical administration prior to routine cataract surgery. Curr Med Res Opin 21(1):93–94
27. Sugioka K et al (2009) Intraocular penetration of sequentially instilled topical moxifloxacin, gatifloxacin, and levofloxacin. Clin Ophthalmol 3:553–557
28. Yagci R et al (2007) Penetration of second-, third-, and fourth-generation topical fluoroquinolone into aqueous and vitreous humour in a rabbit endophthalmitis model. Eye (Lond) 21(7): 990–994
29. Alfonso EC et al (1990) In vitro toxicity of gentamicin to corneal epithelial cells. Cornea 9(1):55–61
30. Baum J (1982) Treatment of bacterial ulcers of the cornea in the rabbit: a comparison of administration by eye drops and subconjunctival injections. Trans Am Ophthalmol Soc 80:369–390
31. Jenkins CD et al (1996) Comparative intraocular penetration of topical and injected cefuroxime. Br J Ophthalmol 80(8):685–688
32. Karpecki P (2009) Besifloxacin ophthalmic suspension 0.6% in patients with bacterial conjunctivitis: a multicenter, prospective, randomized, double-masked, vehicle-controlled, 5-day efficacy and safety study. Clin Ther 31(3):514–526
33. Proksch JW et al (2009) Ocular pharmacokinetics of besifloxacin following topical administration to rabbits, monkeys, and humans. J Ocul Pharmacol Ther 25(4):335–344
34. Sanders ME et al (2011) Comparison of besifloxacin, gatifloxacin, and moxifloxacin against strains of *Pseudomonas aeruginosa* with different quinolone susceptibility patterns in a rabbit model of keratitis. Cornea 30(1):83–90
35. Sanders ME et al (2009) Efficacy of besifloxacin in a rabbit model of methicillin-resistant *Staphylococcus aureus* keratitis. Cornea 28(9):1055–1060
36. Pankey GA (2005) Tigecycline. J Antimicrob Chemother 56(3):470–480
37. Moellering RC (2003) Linezolid: the first oxazolidinone antimicrobial. Ann Intern Med 138(2):135–142
38. Ekdawi NS (2005) Topical linezolid in *Streptococcus pneumoniae* corneal ulcer model in rabbits. Invest Ophthalmol Vis Sci 46(5):4910
39. Saleh M (2010) Ocular penetration of topically applied linezolid in a rabbit model. J Cataract Refract Surg 36(3):488–492
40. Baldwin CM, Lyseng-Williamson KA, Keam SJ (2008) Meropenem: a review of its use in the treatment of serious bacterial infections. Drugs 68(6):803–838
41. Manav C (2004) Comparison of intravitreal ceftazidime and meropenem in treatment of experimental pseudomonal posttraumatic endophthalmitis in a rabbit model. J Appl Res 4(2):337–345
42. Schauersberger J et al (1999) Penetration and decay of meropenem into the human aqueous humor and vitreous. J Ocul Pharmacol Ther 15(5):439–445
43. Moellering RC Jr, Wennersten C, Weinberg AN (1971) Synergy of penicillin and gentamicin against *Enterococci*. J Infect Dis 124(Suppl):S207–S209
44. Winstanley TG, Hastings JG (1990) Synergy between penicillin and gentamicin against enterococci. J Antimicrob Chemother 25(4):551–560
45. Friedland IR, Klugman KP (1992) Failure of chloramphenicol therapy in penicillin-resistant pneumococcal meningitis. Lancet 339(8790):405–408
46. Sueke H et al (2010) An in vitro investigation of synergy or antagonism between antimicrobial combinations against isolates from bacterial keratitis. Invest Ophthalmol Vis Sci 51(8): 4151–4155
47. Kearns VR, Williams RL (2009) Drug delivery systems for the eye. Expert Rev Med Devices 6(3):277–290
48. Behar-Cohen F (2002) Drug delivery systems to target the anterior segment of the eye: fundamental bases and clinical applications. J Fr Ophtalmol 25(5):537–544
49. Luchs JI, Nelinson DS, Macy JI (2010) Efficacy of hydroxypropyl cellulose ophthalmic inserts (LACRISERT) in subsets of patients with dry eye syndrome: findings from a patient registry. Cornea 29(12):1417–1427

Heredity of Keratoconus

3

Colin E. Willoughby and Judith Lechner

Introduction

Advances in the genetic analyses of the corneal dystrophies were a key driver in the IC3D Classification of Corneal Dystrophies. The genetic dissection of corneal dystrophies identified both genetic heterogeneity, when different genes (cytokeratin 3 and cytokeratin 12) can cause an identical corneal phenotype (Meesmann dystrophy) and phenotypic heterogeneity, when different mutations in a single gene (transforming growth factor, beta-induced or *TGFBI*) cause different corneal phenotypes (Reis-Bucklers corneal dystrophy, Thiel-Behnke corneal dystrophy, type 1 and 2 granular corneal dystrophy and lattice type 1) [1]. Genetic insights into the pathogenesis and understanding of keratoconus have been more modest. Keratoconus accounts for 25% of the 2,500 corneal transplants performed annually in the UK and a similar proportion of the 32,000 grafts performed in the USA every year [2]. The use of corneal intrastromal ring segments and collagen cross-linking are now established in the clinical management of keratoconus. The ability to develop new therapeutic options and to improve existing treatments depends on understanding the pathogenesis of keratoconus. Despite the visual and social impact of keratoconus, its underlying biochemical and cellular basis is poorly understood. However, there is a body of evidence to support an underlying genetic basis for this disease.

C.E. Willoughby (✉) • J. Lechner
School of Medicine, Dentistry and Biomedical Sciences,
Centre for Vision and Vascular Science, Queen's University Belfast,
Royal Victoria Hospital,
Grosvenor Road, Belfast BT12 6BA, UK
e-mail: c.willoughby@qub.ac.uk; jlechner01@qub.ac.uk

T. Reinhard, F. Larkin (eds.), *Corneal Disease*,
DOI 10.1007/978-3-642-28747-3_3, © Springer-Verlag Berlin Heidelberg 2013

Is Keratoconus a Heritable or Genetic Disease?

There are numerous studies which support a role of heredity in the development of keratoconus. There is a strong familial predisposition in keratoconus development. A positive family history is reported by 6–10% of patients [3–5] or even as high as 23.5% in some populations [6]. The estimated prevalence of keratoconus in first-degree relatives is 3.34% or 15–67 times higher than general population prevalence of 0.23–0.05% [7]. In most published studies, the inheritance pattern of keratoconus is autosomal dominant with incomplete penetrance or variable expressivity [4, 8–12]. Low expressivity forms of keratoconus, referred to as subclinical or 'forme fruste' keratoconus, can be detected using corneal topography in the relatives of keratoconus patients [13, 14]. Studies in consanguineous populations strongly suggest the existence of recessive forms of keratoconus [15, 16]. Additionally, in a genetic modelling study in a multi-ethnicity population, a major recessive genetic defect was the most parsimonious genetic model [7]. X-linked inheritance has been reported rarely [17]. The role of heredity in disease development can be implied from twin studies, with a higher concordance rate between monozygotic versus dizygotic twins and non-twins, supportive of a genetic aetiology rather than environmental effects. Ideally, the zygosity should be confirmed using genetic typing. Most studies employing corneal topography support the concept of greater concordance between monozygotic twins and hence the role of heredity in keratoconus development [18–20]. Keratoconus commonly presents as an isolated sporadic condition but can be associated with a variety of single-gene disorders and chromosomal aneuploidies [3]. The increased prevalence of keratoconus in trisomy 21, 0.5–15% or 10–300 times the normal population prevalence, has implicated chromosome 21 as a positional candidate for the causative gene [21, 22].

Two approaches have been used to determine the genetic basis of keratoconus: candidate gene sequencing and genetic mapping. Candidate genes are identified based on functional or biological information which makes them plausible agents in the disease pathogenesis or with genetic mapping and linkage analysis also known as positional cloning. Genetic mapping is a powerful technique as no assumptions are made about the causative gene and therefore genes of unknown function or deemed unlikely to be related to disease pathophysiology can be identified.

Mutational Screening of Candidate Genes in Keratoconus

Visual System Homeobox Gene 1 (VSX1)

Héon et al. [23] used linkage analysis to map a major gene for posterior polymorphous corneal dystrophy-1 (PPCD1) to chromosome 20p11-q11 and subsequently identified mutations in the visual system homeobox gene 1 (*VSX1*) in PPCD1 and keratoconus. Héon et al. [24] inferred a role for *VSX1* in keratoconus pathogenesis as earlier case reports had documented the co-existence of PPCD and keratoconus. Following this original publication, there has been debate in the literature about the significance of *VSX1* mutations in keratoconus. Some authors have questioned the role of *VSX1* in keratoconus because of a failure to detect *VSX1* mutations in some keratoconus cohorts [25–27], coupled with the fact that the *VSX1* knockout mouse did not have a corneal phenotype on histological analysis [28] and the initial report of *VSX1* expression in the normal adult human cornea [29] could not be replicated in subsequent studies on normal and keratoconic corneas [24, 30, 31]. However, *VSX1* expression has been detected in the murine cornea [32, 33] and was recently reported in the human neonatal cornea [34]. *VSX1* has a role in corneal wound healing participating in the differentiation of corneal keratocytes into myofibroblasts [35] which may be relevant to the pathogenesis of keratoconus.

VSX1 belongs to the 'paired-like' subfamily of homeodomain (HD) proteins. The homeodomain in this family is related to the homeodomain (HD) of the Drosophila 'paired' protein. *VSX1* also contains a highly conserved CVC domain, essential for transcriptional regulation, which takes its name from the genes it was originally identified in: mouse *Chx10*, goldfish *Vsx1*, and *Caenorhabditis elegans Ceh-10* genes [29]. *VSX1* is expressed in embryonic craniofacial, adult retina and the cornea. The 'paired-like' homeodomain proteins have been implicated in craniofacial and ocular development [28, 29, 32, 36]. Previously, *VSX1* was reported as a five-exon gene but two novel exons downstream of the original *VSX1* gene sequence have been identified. *VSX1* is now known to consist of seven exons with a complex splicing pattern producing a total of six transcripts [34].

In order to determine pathogenicity in any gene-sequencing study, researchers must determine whether the detected sequence variants are deleterious and disease-causing, that is a mutation. Pathological sequence variants or mutations are not seen in ethnically matched controls (and if present, the variant is a polymorphism) and if the condition is familial, segregation of the variant should be seen within the family (affected family members carry the mutation and unaffected have a normal sequence). Pathogenicity can also be predicted based on amino acid conservation, biochemistry and structure using a range of computational tools. The ultimate test is to demonstrate a functional and pathological effect from the sequence variant in disease pathogenesis. Héon et al. [24] reported a functional impact of the Arg166Trp *VSX1* mutation associated with keratoconus on homeodomain binding.

A number of studies [24–27, 37–44] have reported the findings from *VSX1* sequencing in keratoconus and identified sequence variants as shown in Table 3.1. Some of these sequence variants were classified as pathogenic mutations, but the data from subsequent studies or a re-assessment of the original data, shows some of these variants are polymorphisms. To date, there have been 12 mutational studies of *VSX1* in keratoconus involving greater than 1,000 patients. A critical appraisal of all reported *VSX1* mutations in keratoconus leaves six sequence variants which are pathological mutations given the available data (see Table 3.1): Leu17Pro, Asn151Ser, Gly160Asp, Gly160Val, Arg166Trp and Gln175His. Across all published studies, mutations in *VSX1* are present in approximately 2–3% of keratoconus patients. *VSX1* represents the only major genetic defect identified to date causing keratoconus. The most commonly reported mutation was Gly160Val, although the

Table 3.1 Reported sequence variants in VSX1 in sporadic and familial keratoconus patients

Mutation	Ethnicity	KC patients screened	Segregation in familial cases	Controls	Author	Author classification	Classification
Leu17Pro	Italian	3/100	Segregated	0/125	Bisceglia et al. [37]	Mutation	Mutation
Asp144Glu	Unspecified	1/63	Not established	0/277[a]	Héon et al. [24]	Polymorphism	Polymorphism
Asp144Glu	Italian	2/80	Not established	0/125	Bisceglia et al. [37]	Mutation	
Asp144Glu	Unspecified	1/100	Sporadic	0/?[b]	Aldave et al. [25]	Polymorphism	
Asp144Glu	Mixed	1/85	Did not segregate	0/50	Liskova et al. [38]	Polymorphism	
Asp144Glu	Slovenian	1/113	Sporadic	1/100	Stabuc-Silih et al. [39]	Polymorphism	
Asp144Glu	Ashkenazi Jew	1 family	Present	1/104	Eran et al. [40]	Mutation	
Asp144Glu	Northern European	1/66	Did not segregate	0/100	Dash [41]	Polymorphism	
Asn151Ser	Korean	1/249	Sporadic	0/208	Mok et al. [42]	Mutation	Mutation
Leu159Met	unspecified	1/63	Not established	0/277	Héon et al. [24]	Mutation	Polymorphism
Leu159Met	unspecified	0/77	Sporadic	1/71	Tang et al. [26]	Polymorphism	
Leu159Met	unspecified	444 individuals from 75 families: 3 affected and 2 unaffected had variant			Tang et al. [26]	Polymorphism	
Gly160Asp	Italian	2/80	Not established	0/125	Bisceglia et al. [37]	Mutation	Mutation
Gly160Asp	Northern European	2/66	Sporadic	0/100	Dash [41]	Potentially Pathogenic	
Gly160Val	Korean	13/249	Sporadic	0/208	Mok et al. [42]	Mutation	Mutation
Arg166Trp	Unspecified	1/63	Sporadic	0/277	Héon et al. [24]	Mutation	Mutation
Gln175His	Northern India	1/66	Sporadic	0/100	Paliwal et al. [43]	Mutation	Mutation
Arg217His	Northern European	1/66	Absent	22/100	Dash [41]	Polymorphism	Polymorphism
Arg217His	Northern India	1/50	Sporadic	0/50	Tanwar et al. [44]	Polymorphism	
Pro237Pro	Northern India	18/50	Sporadic	15/50	Tanwar et al. [44]	Polymorphism	Polymorphism

His244Arg	Unspecified	1/63	Segregated	2/277	Héon et al. [24]	Polymorphism	Polymorphism
His244Arg	Unspecified	444 individuals from 75 families: 3 affected and 2 unaffected had variant			Tang et al. [26]	Polymorphism	
Pro247Arg	Italian	1/80	Segregated	0/125	Bisceglia et al. [37]	Mutation	Polymorphism
Pro247Arg	Mixed	0/85	–	1/50	Liskova et al. [38]	Polymorphism	

[a]Seen in 1/90 primary open-angle glaucoma cases

[b]Number of controls screened not specified and variant previously reported in one control sample [75]

data was skewed by one study in which Gly160Val mutations were seen in 13/249 of sporadic Korean keratoconic patients [42].

From the available data, the pathogenicity and hence classification of Gly160Asp and Asp144Glu can be debated. Gly160Asp was seen in four unrelated keratoconus patients from Northern Europe and Italy in two independent studies and therefore accounts for 17.4% of *VSX1* mutations in keratoconus. Héon et al. [24] initially reported the segregation of Gly160Asp with posterior polymorphous corneal dystrophy and failed to detect this sequence variant in 277 control individuals, although did report that the glycine residue at position 160 was not highly conserved across species. Biscegali et al. [37] detected Gly160Asp in two families with keratoconus. In one family, segregation was not present as Gly160Asp was detected in one family member with keratoconus, but was only seen in 2/4 family members with topographically suspected keratoconus. In the second family, Gly160Asp was present as a compound heterozygote with Leu17Pro in a patient with keratoconus. The Leu17Pro *VSX1* sequence variant was present in two other Italian families in this study. Segregation was demonstrated in one family; however, the patient from the second family was essentially a sporadic case. Leu17Pro was not seen in 125 control individuals and from the evidence appears pathogenic in its own right. Therefore, the role of Gly160Asp in the compound heterozygote state (Gly160Asp/Leu17Pro) is difficult to ascertain, especially as two other family members had Leu17Pro alone and had evidence of topographically suspected keratoconus. Dash et al. [41] detected Gly160Asp in two sporadic keratoconic patients from Northern Europe which was not seen in 100 control individuals. This author reported that the Gly160 residue is not well conserved across species and was predicted to be a benign variant using bioinformatics modelling. Consequently, the pathogenicity of Gly160Asp can be debated. Gly160Asp is unlikely to represent a rare polymorphism as the glycine 160 amino acid is invariant in 433 controls (combined data across all keratoconus studies). Including the data from Héon et al. [24] on this variant in PPCD, the glycine 160 residue is invariant in 710 controls. Gly160Asp may represent a genetic modifier as compound heterozygotes, as Gly160Asp in association with Leu17Pro [37] and Pro247Arg [24] had clinically more severe corneal phenotypes, suggesting it has an additive effect on keratoconus pathogenesis.

Asp144Glu was reported as a mutation in keratoconus in one study [37], but has been seen in controls [39, 40] and did not segregate in familial keratoconus in two studies [38, 41]. Héon et al. [24] detected Asp144Glu in two family members affected with keratoconus and PPCD and in 1/90 glaucoma patients. The data in the literature suggests Asp144Glu is a polymorphism. Eran et al. [40] proposed Asp144Glu may confer a degree of susceptibility to keratoconus as the residue is highly conserved across species. Additionally, the author reported a higher frequency of the Asp144Glu substitution in keratoconus patients versus the control population. Similarly, Mok et al. [42] reported a higher frequency of an intronic variant (IVS1–11*a) in keratoconus patients versus controls increasing the risk of keratoconus. Some *VSX1* sequence variants (Gly160Asp; Asp144Glu; IVS1–11*a) may not be directly pathogenic but confer a susceptibility to disease development.

Superoxide Dismutase 1 (SOD1)

SOD1 was identified as a potential candidate gene in keratoconus due to its location on chromosome 21 and due to the fact that there is a higher prevalence of keratoconus in Down syndrome patients [21, 22]. Udar et al. [45] performed mutational analysis of SOD1 in 15 unrelated individuals with a family history of keratoconus. A seven base pair deletion in intron 2 of *SOD1* (IVS2+50del7) was detected in two unrelated individuals with familial keratoconus, and absent from 156 control individuals. Segregation could be assessed in one family. RT-PCR on RNA extracted from the blood of one affected individual carrying the *SOD1* intronic mutation and two control individuals showed the presence of two additional major splice variants associated with the intronic mutation. These splice variants lack either exon 2 or both exon 2 and 3 and are predicted to alter SOD1 levels and function [46]. SOD1 binds copper and zinc in a complex, CuZn-SOD, which is an essential antioxidant in the cornea [47]. Following this study, Udar et al. [48] reported that both families harbouring the *SOD1* intronic deletion had distinct haplotypes suggesting the mutation developed independently in these two families. A second study in 113 Slovenian patients with sporadic and familial keratoconus failed to detect pathogenic variants in *SOD1* associated with keratoconus [39]. In conclusion, the role of *SOD1* mutations in keratoconus has not been firmly established.

Interleukin 1 (IL1) Superfamily

Interleukin 1 (*IL1*) has been proposed as a candidate gene for keratoconus [49]. Keratocyte apoptosis and stromal thinning in keratoconic corneas is triggered by the epithelial release of interleukin 1 (IL1) [49, 50]. Kim et al. [49] investigated 12 polymorphic sites in the *IL1* gene cluster in 100 unrelated Korean keratoconus patients. Two SNPs in the promoter region of *IL1B* were significantly different between patient and control groups: −511 (rs16944) and −31 (rs1143627). The combination of the alleles (haplotype) −31*C and −511*T, was associated with an additive increased risk for keratoconus. These two promoter variants and the *IL1B*-31 T/-511 C haplotype are associated with regulation of IL1α and IL1β production [49]. Interleukins are central modulators of the response to corneal injury and there is evidence they play a role in keratoconus.

Collagen Genes

Disruption of *COL8A1* and *COL8A2* in a knockout mouse model resulted in corneal thinning: keratoglobus [51]. *COL8A2* is also mutated in both PPCD and Fuch's endothelial corneal dystrophy [52]. Aldave et al. [53] screened *COL8A2* and *COL8A1* in 50 unrelated patients with keratoconus but failed to detect any pathological variants. Mutations in type IV collagens cause Alport syndrome, a triad of nephropathy, sensorineural deafness and eye features which include anterior lenticonus, perimacular flecks, PPCD and keratoconus [54]. *COL4A3* has been implicated in the pathogenesis of PPCD [33] and both *COL4A3* and *COL4A4* are differentially expressed in keratoconus [55]. Sequencing *COL4A3* and *COL4A4* in 104 unrelated Slovenian patients with keratoconus did not detect mutations [56]. There were significant differences in the genotypes of seven previously reported polymorphisms in *COL4A3* and *COL4A4* between keratoconic patients and controls but further studies in different populations are required to establish the role of these genes in keratoconus.

Genetic Mapping in Keratoconus

With genetic mapping, the chromosomal position or locus associated with the disease is first identified by typing genetic markers and performing linkage analysis. Candidate genes within the disease interval are then prioritised for sequencing based on gene function and biological data. The LOD score (or logarithm_{10} of odds) is a statistical test used for linkage analysis. Positive LOD scores support linkage, whereas negative LOD scores indicate that linkage is less likely. A LOD score of greater than 3.0 is considered strong evidence for linkage giving a 1,000:1 chance that the linkage did not occur by chance alone. A LOD score of less than −2.0 indicates a significant absence of linkage; those between 2.0 and 3.0 are suggestive of linkage, whereas those between −2.0 and +2.0 are uninformative. For sufficient statistical power, large pedigrees give more information for genetic mapping. Standard LOD score linkage analysis is called parametric as it requires a precise genetic model which takes into account the mode of inheritance, gene frequencies and penetrance. Non-parametric linkage analysis uses a model-free method in which only affected individuals are considered. Shared alleles or loci are identified and a non-parametric LOD (NPL) score is generated. The threshold of significance for a NPL is not as defined as the parametric LOD score and significance is usually expressed as a genome wide p value.

Two initial studies of gene mapping in keratoconus [8, 57] used founder populations, in order to increase the power to detect genetic determinants of keratoconus [58]. Fullerton et al. [57] applied a genome-wide identity-by-descent approach in a genetically isolated population from Tasmania in order to circumvent the rarity of large families with keratoconus for mapping and to avoid making assumptions about the genetic model or inheritance pattern. An association of microsatellite markers on chromosome 20 identified a putative locus at 20q12 for keratoconus in related Tasmanian patients. The conserved minimal chromosomal haplotype spanned 3.5 cM between microsatellite markers D20S119 and D20S888, although no underlying genetic defect was identified and a nearby putative candidate gene *MMP-9* was excluded. Utilising the familial keratoconus prevalence of 19% in northern Finland [4], a genome-wide linkage study in 20 Finnish families with autosomal dominant keratoconus mapped a keratoconus disease locus to chromosome 16q [8]. This was the first reported genome-wide linkage study in keratoconus and utilised multiple, small nuclear families, each having two or more affected members without other associated genetic disease. Depending on the analysis model, a maximum multipoint LOD score of 4.10 (parametric) and 3.27 (non-parametric) were obtained. The disease locus was a 6.9 cM interval on chr16q22.3-q23.1 between genetic markers D16S2624 and D16S3090. However, no causative gene has been identified to date. Applying a similar approach in southern Italian keratoconus patients, a region of putative but not statistically significant linkage was reported close to the Finnish locus identified by Tyynismaa et al. [8] at 16q23 (106 cM) [59].

Following these initial linkage studies, a number of authors reported the results of genome-wide linkage screens using microsatellite markers regularly spaced across the genome in large autosomal dominant Caucasian families. Hughes et al. [9] identified a keratoconus locus on chromosome 15q22–24 in a large three-generation Northern Irish family (16 affected and 14 unaffected individuals), affected by combined early onset autosomal dominant anterior polar cataract and clinically severe keratoconus. A maximum 2-point LOD score of 8.13 was found at *IREB2* and the disease interval was 6.5 Mb flanked by *CYP11A* and D15S211. The disease interval is exceedingly gene rich, containing approximately 95 known or predicted genes. No pathogenic variants were detected in the coding regions of four positional candidate genes for keratoconus and cataract: *cathepsin H gene* (*CTSH*), *cellular retinoic acid binding protein 1 gene* (*CRABP1*), *iron-responsive element binding protein 2* gene (*IREB2*) and the *Ras guanine nucleotide releasing factor gene* (*RASGRF1*). Dash et al. [60] refined the linkage region in this family to an interval of approximately 5.5 Mb flanked by the *MAN2C1* gene and the D15S211 microsatellite marker on chromosome 15q. This excluded a further 28 candidate genes and direct sequencing of a further 23 candidate genes failed to detect a causative mutation. Recently, using a newly established sequencing technique, the whole 5.5 Mb linkage region was captured on a custom-designed DNA array, amplified and interrogated with next-generation or massively parallel sequencing. Work is ongoing to elucidate the genetic basis of keratoconus in this family [61].

The results of a genome-wide linkage screen were reported in two other Caucasian families with autosomal dominant keratoconus [10, 11]. Firstly, a genome-wide linkage study in an Italian pedigree, consisting of 11 family members in two-generation manifesting autosomal dominant keratoconus, identified a locus on chromosome 3p14-q13 with a maximum LOD score of 3.09. The linkage interval was large, spanning the centromere of chromosome 3, between microsatellite markers D3S1600 and D3S1278 covering 53 Mb of DNA, of which approximately 4.5 Mb was centromeric DNA [10]. No other families have been linked to this keratoconus disease locus. The region contains over 100 genes, including the gene for the human alpha1 (VIII) chain of type VIII collagen, *COL8A1*, which is highly expressed in the cornea. However, no mutations were detected in this attractive potential candidate gene in this family and *COL8A1* was sequenced in a subsequent study of 50 unrelated keratoconus patients and no pathogenic mutations were detected [53]. Secondly, a genome-wide linkage study in a four-generation Caucasian family identified a keratoconus disease locus on chromosome 5q14.3-q21.1 [11]. This family was previously mapped to chromosome 21 with a multipoint LOD score of 2.4 for markers on 21q [62]. The pedigree was complex as it involved two families connected by a mating between two affected individuals but there was no evidence of a common ancestry. Due to the pedigree complexity, a number of data analysis strategies were employed and fine mapping following the initial analysis identified a linkage peak between microsatellite markers D5S2499 and D5S495 on chromosome 5q14.1-q21.3 with a LOD score of 3.53. This is a 6 cM region containing 8.2 Mb of DNA. This locus was replicated by Bisceglia et al. [59] who performed a genome-wide microsatellite scan in 133 individuals from southern Italy (77 affected and 59 unaffected) belonging to 25 families. Bisceglia et al. [59] identified a large region, spanning 70 cM, on chromosome 5q with a significant non-parametric linkage (NPL) analysis LOD score ($p<0.05$). At the boundaries of this interval were two higher peaks of greater significance ($p<0.01$). One of these fell in 5q21.2 (NPL 2.73, $p=0.003669$) overlapping with the region, between 100 and 120 cM, reported by Tang et al. [11]. No causative gene has been reported to date but this is the only keratoconus locus which has been convincingly replicated in two independent datasets and implicates this genomic region as a key locus involved in the genetic basis of keratoconus.

Most linkage studies in keratoconus have been performed in Caucasian families under a dominant inheritance model or in isolated populations where genetic heterogeneity is minimised. To address this, Hutchings et al. [12] performed a genome-wide scan in an outbred population of mixed ethnicity (Caucasian, Arab and Caribbean African) and mapped a new locus for keratoconus to chromosome 2p24. There was no clear evidence of non-parametric linkage, and in most families keratoconus was inherited in a dominant manner with incomplete penetrance. Using a dominant linkage model, a significant parametric LOD score of 5.13 was obtained. The disease haplotype segregated in 17/28 or 60% of families. Linkage to all other known keratoconus loci, at that time, on chromosomes 3, 16, 20 and 21 was excluded. The new keratoconus locus on 2p24 was a relatively small region of 1.69 Mb flanked by microsatellite markers D2S305 and D2S2372. The region was refined to 0.9 Mb in one family and the disease interval contained eight known genes and ten predicted genes. However, no mutations were identified. In a similar manner and in order to increase genetic heterogeneity, Li et al. [63] employed a two-stage genome-wide linkage scan in 110 white and Hispanic sib-pairs using a non-parametric method in an attempt to identify susceptibility genes for keratoconus. The most significant signal (LOD=4.5) was detected at the telomere of chromosome 9q34 (159 cM) in all pedigrees (white and Hispanic). Other putative loci were detected with non-significant LOD scores. The putative loci at 14q11 and 5q32-q33 reported by Li et al. [63] were observed in a subsequent study but again failed to reach significance [59]. However, the fact that these putative loci with suggestive linkage were independently detected in two datasets cannot be discounted and these genomic regions may be implicated in the development of keratoconus. Two potential keratoconus candidate genes in 14q11 were highlighted by these authors [59, 63]; *APEX1* and *CIDEB*, but there have been no subsequent reports describing the sequencing of these genes. The *APEX1* gene encodes for APEX nuclease (multifunctional DNA repair enzyme) 1, a DNA repair enzyme which is expressed in the normal and keratoconic cornea. The *cell death-inducing DFFA-like effector b* (*CIDEB*) gene is expressed in the keratoconic cornea and is involved in apoptosis which is increased in keratoconus [47, 64]. Recently, Liskova et al. [65] identified a keratoconus locus on chromosome 14q24.3 using a genome-wide single-nucleotide polymorphism (SNP) DNA chip in six multiethnic families with three to five members affected by keratoconus. The strongest area of linkage was between SNP marker rs1074501 and rs755212 which under a dominant model of inheritance yielded identical LOD scores of 3.58. The interval is 2.8 Mb and includes the transcription factor visual system homeobox 2 gene (*VSX2/ CHX10*), which is involved in eye development and when mutated causes a spectrum of ocular disorder, in particular, non-syndromic microphthalmia/anophthalmia. Mutational screening of *VSX2* was negative and further analysis is ongoing. Interestingly, human *VSX1* is homologous with goldfish *Vsx2* and mouse *Chx10* proteins. Although not in the immediate vicinity of the area at 14q11 identified previously [59, 63], this is secondary evidence of a potential genetic effect originating from this general region on chromosome 14.

In a study assessing Ecuadorian families with autosomal dominant keratoconus, 18 families were identified and in one large keratoconus family, there was evidence of linkage on chromosome 13q32 with a maximum multipoint parametric LOD score of 4.1 and multipoint non-parametric linkage LOD score of 3.2 [27]. The family was typed using a genome-wide SNP array which identified a 5.6 Mb disease interval between the SNPs rs9516572 and rs3825523 on 13q32 that contained 23 known genes. The underlying genetic defect has not been identified to date. Using a genome-wide SNP array in a large Australian pedigree apparently manifesting autosomal dominant keratoconus identified two regions of linkage: 1p36.23–36.21 and 8q13.1-q21.11. The individual LOD score for these loci were 1.9, respectively; however, concurrent analysis of both loci suggested digenic linkage with a two-locus LOD score of 3.4. The linkage peak on chromosome 1 covered 7.1 Mb from SNP rs966134 to rs2092504 (14.2–27.645 cM) and the larger chromosome 8 peak covered 13.8 Mb between SNPs rs949988 and rs1021157 (77.0–90.0 cM). All affected individuals carried both disease haplotypes but family members with only one disease haplotype were normal. Five candidate genes expressed in the cornea within the disease haplotype (*ENO1, PLOD1, UBIAD1,* SPSB1and *TCEB1)* were sequenced but no mutations were detected [66]. This was the first report of digenic inheritance in keratoconus. In digenic inheritance, the phenotype results from a genetic defect in two different genes and the combination of both defects is required to cause the disease. Individuals with a mutation in only one gene are therefore normal. There are a number of ocular disorders associated with digenic inheritance: retinitis pigmentosa and primary open-angle glaucoma [67]. All reported loci associated with keratoconus are summarised in Table 3.2.

Genetics of Keratoconus – Mendelian or Complex?

Human disease phenotypes are classified as either simple Mendelian disorders or complex conditions. Simple or Mendelian phenotypes follow distinctive patterns of inheritance (autosomal dominant or recessive, or X-linked) and are monogenic, in

Table 3.2 Chromosomal loci associated with keratoconus

Study group	Chromosomal locus	Reference
Australian family	1p36.23-36.21	Bourdon et al. [66]
	8q13.1-q21.11	
28 families from Europe and West Indies	2p24	Hutchings et al. [12]
Italian family	3p14-q13	Brancati et al. [10]
Caucasian family	5q14.3-q21.1	Tang [11]
110 white and Hispanic sibling-pairs	9q34	Li et al. [63]
1 family from Ecuador	13q32	Gajecka [27]
6 Multiethnic families	14q24.3	Liskova et al. [65]
Northern Irish family	15q22.33-q24.2	Hughes et al. [9]
20 Finish families	16q22.3-q23.1	Tyynismaa [8]
8 individuals from Tasmania	20q12	Fullerton et al. [57]

which only one particular genetic variant or allele is required to cause the phenotype. In contrast, complex disorders result from a combination of factors, both genetic and environmental. In complex genetic disorders, the different alleles of particular genes increase the probability of a phenotype or condition to develop but not with absolute certainty. These genetic factors are known as susceptibility genes. Some genetic variants in *VSX1*, *COL4A3*, *COL4A4* and *IL1B*, as discussed earlier, may act as susceptibility variants predisposing to the development of keratoconus [41, 49, 56]. Between the genetic extremes of rare monogenic and common polygenic or complex diseases lie oligogenic disorders requiring mutations in more than one gene to cause the phenotype [68]. In contrast to polygenic traits, oligogenic disorders are primarily genetic, but require the synergistic interaction of mutant alleles at a small number of loci. There is a conceptual continuum between classical monogenic Mendelian and complex traits bridged by oligogenic disorders.

The genetic mapping studies in keratoconus (see Table 3.2) demonstrate the importance of genetic determinants in its development, but the lack of consistently mapped chromosomal loci in these studies indicates genetic heterogeneity. If keratoconus is considered a pure dominant Mendelian disorder, then incomplete penetrance and variable expressivity could explain variation in the clinical phenotype (unilateral or bilateral disease, variable age of onset, variable progression and presence of subclinical forms). Similarly, this clinical variability could be explained by a complex, multiple susceptibility gene model. The clinical variability and the evidence that keratoconus is linked to multiple chromosomal regions is consistent with an oligogenic model and even a polygenic/multiple susceptibility gene model. In addition, the genetic heterogeneity could support an oligogenic model in which mutations in several different genes, involved in related pathways, may act on common targets responsible for the disease. Genome-wide association studies (GWAS) are used to investigate common, complex diseases [69].

GWAS studies may be a more appropriate methodology to determine the genetic basis of keratoconus. With this technique, genetic variants or SNPs from across the genome are typed using DNA microarrays in cases and controls. The aim is to detect genetic variants more commonly seen in the cases than controls, hence 'associated' with the disease, and so identifies an area of the genome for further analysis [69]. Using this approach in keratoconus patients from Australia and Northern Ireland, Burdon et al. [70] identified SNPs in hepatocyte growth factor (*HGF*) associated with keratoconus. Similar but larger studies have recently detected genetic variants in *COL5A1* and *ZNF469*, associated with central corneal thickness, which might be relevant to keratoconus genetics [71, 72]. Brittle cornea syndrome (BCS) is characterised by blue sclerae, corneal rupture, keratoconus or keratoglobus, exaggerated elasticity of the skin and joint hypermobility. Mutations in *zinc finger protein 469* (*ZNF469*) cause BCS [73] and this gene has not been evaluated in keratoconus to date. Further GWA studies in keratoconus are required involving larger cohorts and collaboration between research groups. A GWAS was recently successful in Fuch's endothelial dystrophy [74] and applying this approach should bring further insights into the genetic basis of keratoconus.

References

1. Weiss JS et al (2008) The IC3D classification of the corneal dystrophies. Cornea 27(Suppl 2):S1–S83
2. Rahman I et al (2009) Penetrating keratoplasty: indications, outcomes, and complications. Eye (Lond) 23(6):1288–1294
3. Rabinowitz YS (1998) Keratoconus. Surv Ophthalmol 42(4):297–319
4. Ihalainen A (1986) Clinical and epidemiological features of keratoconus genetic and external factors in the pathogenesis of the disease. Acta Ophthalmol Suppl 178:1–64
5. Edwards M, McGhee CN, Dean S (2001) The genetics of keratoconus. Clin Experiment Ophthalmol 29(6):345–351
6. Owens H, Gamble G (2003) A profile of keratoconus in New Zealand. Cornea 22(2):122–125
7. Wang Y et al (2000) Genetic epidemiological study of keratoconus: evidence for major gene determination. Am J Med Genet 93(5):403–409
8. Tyynismaa H (2002) A locus for autosomal dominant keratoconus: linkage to 16q22.3-q23.1 in Finnish families. Invest Ophthalmol Vis Sci 43(10):3160–3164
9. Hughes AE et al (2003) Familial keratoconus with cataract: linkage to the long arm of chromosome 15 and exclusion of candidate genes. Invest Ophthalmol Vis Sci 44(12):5063–5066
10. Brancati F et al (2004) A locus for autosomal dominant keratoconus maps to human chromosome 3p14-q13. J Med Genet 41(3):188–192
11. Tang YG (2005) Genomewide linkage scan in a multigeneration Caucasian pedigree identifies a novel locus for keratoconus on chromosome 5q14.3-q21.1. Genet Med 7(6):397–405
12. Hutchings H et al (2005) Identification of a new locus for isolated familial keratoconus at 2p24. J Med Genet 42(1):88–94
13. Levy D et al (2004) Videokeratographic anomalies in familial keratoconus. Ophthalmology 111(5):867–874
14. Rabinowitz YS, Garbus J, McDonnell PJ (1990) Computer-assisted corneal topography in family members of patients with keratoconus. Arch Ophthalmol 108(3):365–371
15. Georgiou T et al (2004) Influence of ethnic origin on the incidence of keratoconus and associated atopic disease in Asians and white patients. Eye (Lond) 18(4):379–383
16. Pearson AR et al (2000) Does ethnic origin influence the incidence or severity of keratoconus? Eye (Lond) 14(Pt 4):625–628

17. Hammerstein W (1971) Significance of the sex ratio in the determination of x-chromosomal heredity demonstrated on the clinical picture of keratoconus. Klin Monbl Augenheilkd 159(5):602–608
18. Bechara SJ, Waring GO 3rd, Insler MS (1996) Keratoconus in two pairs of identical twins. Cornea 15(1):90–93
19. Parker J et al (1996) Videokeratography of keratoconus in monozygotic twins. J Refract Surg 12(1):180–183
20. Owens H, Watters GA (1995) Keratoconus in monozygotic twins in New Zealand. Clin Experiment Ophthalmol 78:125–129
21. Shapiro MB, France TD (1985) The ocular features of Down's syndrome. Am J Ophthalmol 99(6):659–663
22. Krachmer JH, Feder RS, Belin MW (1984) Keratoconus and related noninflammatory corneal thinning disorders. Surv Ophthalmol 28(4):293–322
23. Heon E et al (1995) Linkage of posterior polymorphous corneal dystrophy to 20q11. Hum Mol Genet 4(3):485–488
24. Héon E et al (2002) VSX1: a gene for posterior polymorphous dystrophy and keratoconus. Hum Mol Genet 11(9):1029–1036
25. Aldave AJ et al (2006) No VSX1 gene mutations associated with keratoconus. Invest Ophthalmol Vis Sci 47(7):2820–2822
26. Tang YG et al (2008) Three VSX1 gene mutations, L159M, R166W, and H244R, are not associated with keratoconus. Cornea 27(2):189–192
27. Gajecka M (2009) Localization of a gene for keratoconus to a 5.6-Mb interval on 13q32. Invest Ophthalmol Vis Sci 50(4):1531–1539
28. Chow RL et al (2004) Control of late off-center cone bipolar cell differentiation and visual signaling by the homeobox gene Vsx1. Proc Natl Acad Sci USA 101(6):1754–1759
29. Semina EV, Mintz-Hittner HA, Murray JC (2000) Isolation and characterization of a novel human paired-like homeodomain-containing transcription factor gene, VSX1, expressed in ocular tissues. Genomics 63(2):289–293
30. Nielsen K et al (2003) Identification of differentially expressed genes in keratoconus epithelium analyzed on microarrays. Invest Ophthalmol Vis Sci 44(6):2466–2476
31. Rabinowitz YS, Dong L, Wistow G (2005) Gene expression profile studies of human keratoconus cornea for NEIBank: a novel cornea-expressed gene and the absence of transcripts for aquaporin 5. Invest Ophthalmol Vis Sci 46(4):1239–1246
32. Chow RL et al (2001) Vsx1, a rapidly evolving paired-like homeobox gene expressed in cone bipolar cells. Mech Dev 109(2):315–322
33. Krafchak CM et al (2005) Mutations in TCF8 cause posterior polymorphous corneal dystrophy and ectopic expression of COL4A3 by corneal endothelial cells. Am J Hum Genet 77(5):694–708
34. Hosseini SM et al (2008) Genetic analysis of chromosome 20-related posterior polymorphous corneal dystrophy: genetic heterogeneity and exclusion of three candidate genes. Mol Vis 14:71–80
35. Barbaro V et al (2006) Expression of VSX1 in human corneal keratocytes during differentiation into myofibroblasts in response to wound healing. Invest Ophthalmol Vis Sci 47(12):5243–5250
36. Mintz-Hittner HA et al (2004) VSX1 (RINX) mutation with craniofacial anomalies, empty sella, corneal endothelial changes, and abnormal retinal and auditory bipolar cells. Ophthalmology 111(4):828–836
37. Bisceglia L et al (2005) VSX1 mutational analysis in a series of Italian patients affected by keratoconus: detection of a novel mutation. Invest Ophthalmol Vis Sci 46(1):39–45
38. Liskova P et al (2007) Molecular analysis of the VSX1 gene in familial keratoconus. Mol Vis 13:1887–1891
39. Stabuc-Silih M et al (2010) Absence of pathogenic mutations in VSX1 and SOD1 genes in patients with keratoconus. Cornea 29(2):172–176
40. Eran P et al (2008) The D144E substitution in the VSX1 gene: a non-pathogenic variant or a disease causing mutation? Ophthalmic Genet 29(2):53–59

41. Dash DP (2009) Mutational screening of VSX1 in keratoconus patients from the European population. Eye (Lond) 24(6):1085–1092
42. Mok JW, Baek SJ, Joo CK (2008) VSX1 gene variants are associated with keratoconus in unrelated Korean patients. J Hum Genet 53(9):842–849
43. Paliwal P et al (2009) A novel VSX1 mutation identified in an individual with keratoconus in India. Mol Vis 15:2475–2479
44. Tanwar M et al (2010) VSX1 gene analysis in keratoconus. Mol Vis 16:2395–2401
45. Udar N et al (2006) SOD1: a candidate gene for keratoconus. Invest Ophthalmol Vis Sci 47(8):3345–3351
46. Kawata A et al (2000) Aberrant splicing of human Cu/Zn superoxide dismutase (SOD1) RNA transcripts. Neuroreport 11(12):2649–2653
47. Chwa M et al (2006) Increased stress-induced generation of reactive oxygen species and apoptosis in human keratoconus fibroblasts. Invest Ophthalmol Vis Sci 47(5):1902–1910
48. Udar N et al (2009) SOD1 haplotypes in familial keratoconus. Cornea 28(8):902–907
49. Kim SH et al (2008) Association of −31 T>C and −511 C>T polymorphisms in the interleukin 1 beta (IL1B) promoter in Korean keratoconus patients. Mol Vis 14:2109–2116
50. Wilson SE et al (1996) Epithelial injury induces keratocyte apoptosis: hypothesized role for the interleukin-1 system in the modulation of corneal tissue organization and wound healing. Exp Eye Res 62(4):325–327
51. Hopfer U et al (2005) Targeted disruption of Col8a1 and Col8a2 genes in mice leads to anterior segment abnormalities in the eye. FASEB J 19(10):1232–1244
52. Biswas S et al (2001) Missense mutations in COL8A2, the gene encoding the alpha2 chain of type VIII collagen, cause two forms of corneal endothelial dystrophy. Hum Mol Genet 10(21):2415–2423
53. Aldave AJ et al (2007) Keratoconus is not associated with mutations in COL8A1 and COL8A2. Cornea 26(8):963–965
54. Chugh KS et al (1993) Hereditary nephritis (Alport's syndrome) – clinical profile and inheritance in 28 kindreds. Nephrol Dial Transplant 8(8):690–695
55. Bochert A (2003) Gene expression in keratoconus. Initial results using DNA microarrays. Ophthalmologe 100(7):545–549
56. Stabuc-Silih M et al (2009) Polymorphisms in COL4A3 and COL4A4 genes associated with keratoconus. Mol Vis 15:2848–2860
57. Fullerton J et al (2002) Identity-by-descent approach to gene localisation in eight individuals affected by keratoconus from north-west Tasmania, Australia. Hum Genet 110(5):462–470
58. Peltonen L, Jalanko A, Varilo T (1999) Molecular genetics of the Finnish disease heritage. Hum Mol Genet 8(10):1913–1923
59. Bisceglia L (2009) Linkage analysis in keratoconus: replication of locus 5q21.2 and identification of other suggestive Loci. Invest Ophthalmol Vis Sci 50(3):1081–1086
60. Dash DP, Silvestri G, Hughes AE (2006) Fine mapping of the keratoconus with cataract locus on chromosome 15q and candidate gene analysis. Mol Vis 12:499–505
61. Willoughby CE et al (2010) Targeted sequence capture and next generation sequencing of a 5 Mb region on chromosome 15q previously linked to keratoconus. Invest Ophthalmol Vis Sci 51:E-Abstract 4644
62. Zu LX (1999) Identification of a putative locus for keratoconus on chromosome 21 (abstract). Am J Hum Genet 65:A31–A161
63. Li X et al (2006) Two-stage genome-wide linkage scan in keratoconus sib pair families. Invest Ophthalmol Vis Sci 47(9):3791–3795
64. Kaldawy RM et al (2002) Evidence of apoptotic cell death in keratoconus. Cornea 21(2):206–209
65. Liskova P et al (2010) Evidence for keratoconus susceptibility locus on chromosome 14: a genome-wide linkage screen using single-nucleotide polymorphism markers. Arch Ophthalmol 128(9):1191–1195
66. Burdon KP et al (2008) Apparent autosomal dominant keratoconus in a large Australian pedigree accounted for by digenic inheritance of two novel loci. Hum Genet 124(4):379–386

67. Ming JE, Muenke M (2002) Multiple hits during early embryonic development: digenic diseases and holoprosencephaly. Am J Hum Genet 71(5):1017–1032
68. Katsanis N (2004) The oligogenic properties of Bardet-Biedl syndrome. Hum Mol Genet 13 Spec No. 1: R65–R71
69. Hirschhorn JN, Daly MJ (2005) Genome-wide association studies for common diseases and complex traits. Nat Rev Genet 6(2):95–108
70. Burdon KP et al (2010) A genome-wide association scan for keratoconus identifies novel candidate genes. Invest Ophthalmol Vis Sci 51: E-Abstract 4646
71. Lu Y et al (2010) Common genetic variants near the brittle cornea syndrome locus ZNF469 influence the blinding disease risk factor central corneal thickness. PLoS Genet 6(5):e1000947
72. Vitart V et al (2010) New loci associated with central cornea thickness include COL5A1, AKAP13 and AVGR8. Hum Mol Genet 19(21):4304–4311
73. Abu A et al (2008) Deleterious mutations in the Zinc-Finger 469 gene cause brittle cornea syndrome. Am J Hum Genet 82(5):1217–1222
74. Baratz KH et al (2010) E2–2 protein and Fuchs's corneal dystrophy. N Engl J Med 363(11):1016–1024
75. Aldave AJ (2005) Candidate gene screening for posterior polymorphous dystrophy. Cornea 24(2):151–155

Advance in Corneal Imaging

4

Antoine Labbé, Alexandre Denoyer,
and Christophe Baudouin

Introduction

Many clinical situations require a precise assessment of corneal structures. However, the resolution of ophthalmic instruments such as the slit-lamp is limited and, for ophthalmologists, it has always been a challenge to evaluate qualitatively and quantitatively the microscopic structures of the cornea. Recently, new imaging techniques have thus been developed to overcome these limitations of light biomicroscopy.

In vivo confocal microscopy (IVCM) is a noninvasive imaging technique that provides high-resolution images of the cornea, the limbus, and the conjunctiva. The usefulness of IVCM to analyze ocular surface structures at a cellular level in normal and pathologic conditions has been largely demonstrated in numerous publications. IVCM actually constitutes an important aid in the diagnosis and the management of infectious keratitis, corneal dystrophies, and for the evaluation of corneal changes after refractive or corneal surgery.

Furthermore, since optical coherence tomography (OCT) was first developed for analysis of the posterior part of the eye, modifications have been made in the technique such that good-resolution images of the anterior segment can be obtained. A large number of AS-OCT applications have been proposed, notably in the field of refractive surgery and corneal graft.

A. Labbé, M.D., Ph.D. • C. Baudouin, M.D., Ph.D. (✉)
Department of Ophthalmology III, Quinze-Vingts National Ophthalmology Hospital,
28 Rue de Charenton, Paris 75012, France
e-mail: chrbaudouin@aol.com

A. Denoyer, M.D.
Department of Ophthalmology III, Quinze-Vingts National Ophthalmology Hospital,
28 Rue de Charenton, Paris 75012, France

T. Reinhard, F. Larkin (eds.), *Corneal Disease*,
DOI 10.1007/978-3-642-28747-3_4,

Like for any new imaging technique, analysis of the images is only possible after a thorough grounding in the semiology. The goal of this chapter is to present a large variety of IVCM and OCT applications in the cornea and anterior segment in order to render this new means of imaging more familiar, making it possible to use these very promising imaging techniques with optimum efficiency.

In Vivo Confocal Microscopy (IVCM)

Despite its use over the last 20 years, it has not been until recently, with new commercially available IVCM devices, that IVCM has become more accessible to clinicians. Combined with high-performance digital imaging, IVCM offers today a non-invasive method of examining the cornea, the limbus or the conjunctiva with possible magnification of up to 400 times.

Principles of Confocal Microscopy

The principle of confocal microscopy was described for the first time by Marvin Minsky back in 1955 while studying brain parenchyma cells. He proposed that the observation (objective) and illumination (condenser) systems be focused in a single point, hence the name "confocal" microscopy. By focusing the observation and illumination system on a single point, light reflected by elements outside the focal point could be excluded, thus increasing image resolution and contrast. The ability of in vivo confocal microscopy to eliminate the light out-of-focus allows up to a few microns axial and lateral resolution. However, the spatial resolution is improved at the cost of a considerable reduction in the field of view (focal point). It is therefore necessary to quickly observe adjacent points and to reconstruct the images in order to allow direct observation of the whole specimen. Different techniques are used to rapidly capture all the points composing the image of the specimen. The Tandem Scanning Confocal Microscope (TSCM) contains a rotating Nipkow disc that has pinholes arranged in Archimedian spirals. This type of in vivo confocal microscope is no longer in production. The Slit Scanning Confocal Microscope (SSCM) uses two optically conjugate scanning optical slits for illumination and detection. SSCM are commercially available from Tomey Corporation (Cambridge, MA, USA), Nidek Technologies (Gamagori, Japan), and Helmut Hund (Wetzlar, Germany). The most recent development in clinical confocal microscopy is the Confocal Laser Scanning Microscope (CLSM) (Heidelberg Retina Tomograph Rostock Cornea Module (HRT-RCM), Heidelberg Engineering, Heidelberg, Germany). Compared to the TSCM and the SSCM that use a white light source, this recently developed confocal microscope uses a 670-nm red wavelength diode laser as a light source. In order to scan the whole specimen, the laser beam is scanned sequentially over each point of the examined area by a set of galvanometer scanning mirrors.

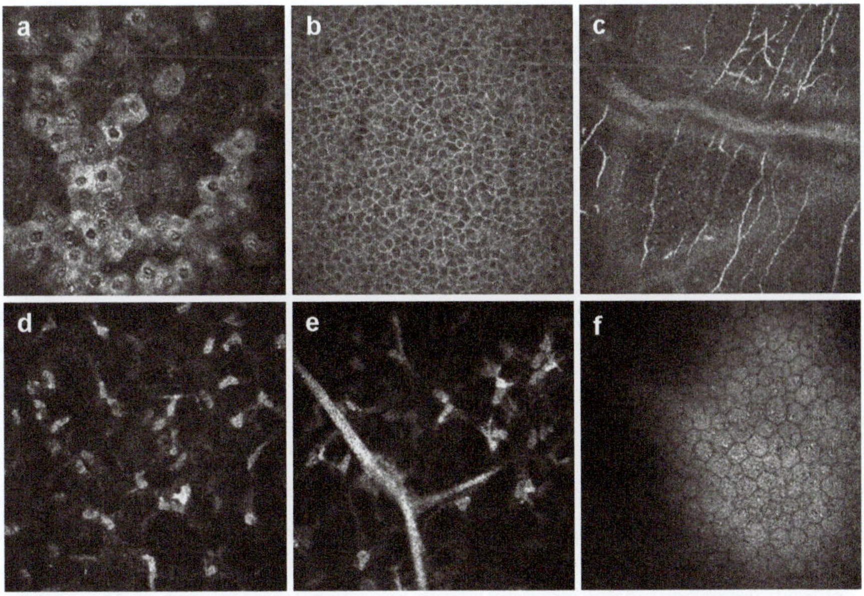

Fig. 4.1 In vivo confocal microscopy (IVCM) images (400×400 μm, Heidelberg Retina Tomograph – Rostock Cornea Module (HRT-RCM)) of the normal cornea. Superficial epithelial cells (**a**). Basal epithelial cells (**b**). Bowman layer with sub-basal nerves (**c**). Anterior stroma with hyper-reflective keratocyte nuclei (**d**). Stromal nerve (**e**). Endothelium (**f**)

The Normal Cornea

With the exception of the normal Descemet membrane, the confocal microscope can provide images of all layers of the cornea. Contrary to conventional microscopy, which provides transverse sections of the tissue, images obtained with IVCM generally consist of optical sections oriented parallel to the surface observed.

The corneal epithelium consists of superficial, intermediate, and basal epithelial cells. Superficial cells appeared as polygonal – often hexagonal – cells with a size up to 50 μm in diameter. The reflectivity is variable but cells undergoing desquamation are characterized by a highly reflective cytoplasm with a visible nuclei and a perinuclear dark halo (Fig. 4.1a). Intermediate epithelial cells or wing cells have a regular form with size up to approximately 20 μm, and are characterized by reflecting cell borders and a dark cytoplasm with rarely visible nuclei. The basal epithelial layer forms a regular mosaic of smaller cells (8–10 μm), with a dark cytoplasm, reflective cell borders, and without visible nuclei (Fig. 4.1b).

The sub-basal nerve plexus is located between Bowman's membrane and the basal epithelium. Sub-basal corneal nerves appear as hyper-reflective, beaded linear structures of 4–8 μm thickness (Fig. 4.1c). Bowman's membrane appears as an amorphous layer of 8–10 μm thickness located between basal cells and the stroma. Only the highly reflective stromal nerves and keratocyte nuclei are visualized on confocal microscopy examination of the normal corneal stroma. Keratocyte nuclei are visible as oval, round or egg-shaped hyper-reflective structures (Fig. 4.1d). Stromal nerves appear as hyper-reflective thick linear structures with sometimes visible dichotomous branches (Fig. 4.1e).

The Descemet membrane is observed as a thin (6–8 μm) amorphous and acellular layer located between the posterior stroma and the endothelium. This layer is not visible in young and normal subjects. The healthy corneal endothelium consists of a monolayer of hexagonal reflective cells arranged regularly in a honeycomb pattern with hypo-reflective cell borders (Fig. 4.1). Although IVCM images of the cornea consist of optical sections oriented parallel to the tissue, cross section may also be obtained. Not only the cornea, but also the conjunctiva and the limbus could be imaged with IVCM [1].

Clinical Applications

The early detection and diagnosis of infectious keratitis and the evaluation of corneal wound healing after refractive surgery or corneal surgery were the first clinical applications of confocal microscopy. With improvement of in vivo confocal microscopes, these clinical applications were developed and new clinical applications have been demonstrated or are under development.

Infectious Keratitis

As an early diagnosis or even a high suspicion of an infective microorganism may lead to treating more rapidly and improve the outcome of infectious keratitis, it represents one of the most important clinical uses of IVCM. However, only the morphology of cells could be used to differentiate cell types and microorganisms with IVCM. As most bacteria have a size below or approaching the resolution limit of IVCM, these microorganisms could not be visualized directly using IVCM unless they presented distinctive features such as a larger size or a filamentous form [2]. Similarly to most bacteria, the virus size does not allow their direct visualization using IVCM. However, structural corneal changes could be observed and monitored in patients with bacterial or viral keratitis and differential diagnosis may benefit from this technique [2].

IVCM can visualize filamentous and yeast fungi within the cornea of patients with FK and may be helpful in managing this disease by providing a rapid diagnosis so that treatment can be initiated earlier [3, 4]. *Fusarium* and *Aspergillus* fungi appear as hyper-reflective interlocking filaments approximately 3–10 μm in width and 200–400 μm in length (Fig. 4.2a–c). Some publications have also reported IVCM images of other fungi such as *Beauveria bassiana*, *Candida Albicans*, *Microsporidia*, *Alternaria alternata*, or *Penicillium* [2].

The clinical diagnosis of *Acanthamoeba* is often difficult because the early clinical presentation is nonspecific. Contrary to viruses and bacteria, the size of *Acanthamoeba* cysts or trophozoites allows their direct visualization using IVCM. Numerous publications have described the use of IVCM as a noninvasive tool to

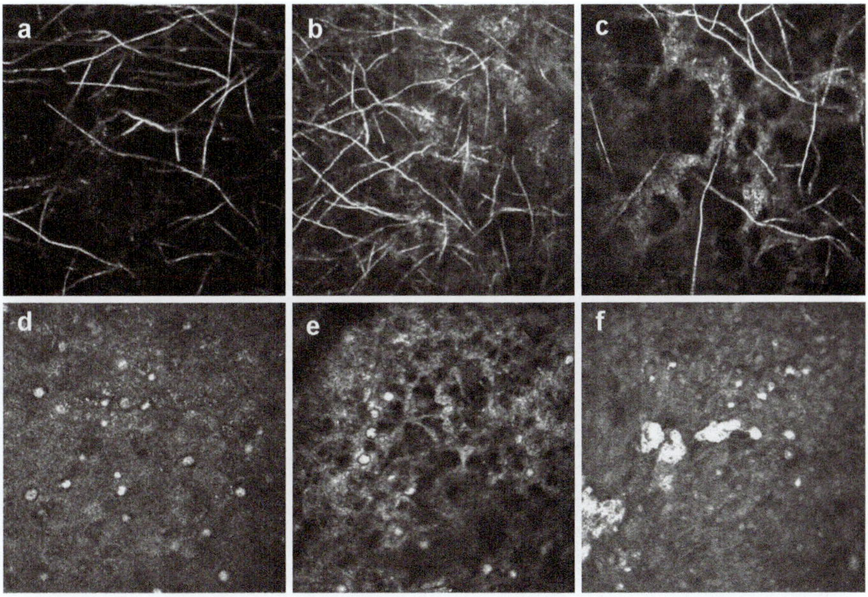

Fig. 4.2 In vivo confocal microscopy (IVCM) images (400×400 μm, Heidelberg Retina Tomograph – Rostock Cornea Module (HRT-RCM)). *Fusarium* fungus appears as hyper-reflective interlocking filaments in the stroma (**a**–**c**). *Acanthamoeba* cysts within the epithelium (**d**) and stroma (**e**). The cysts are observed as round hyper-reflective structures with sometimes a double-wall appearance. *Acanthamoeba* trophozoites appear as multiform hyper-reflective structures within the corneal epithelium (**f**)

diagnose *Acanthamoeba* keratitis (AK) [2, 4]. IVCM can show four signs of AK: cysts, trophozoites, the classic keratoneuritis, and the intrastromal cavities seen during the late stages of the disease. *Acanthamoeba* cysts are observed with IVCM in the epithelium or the stroma as spherical, round, ovoid, pear- or egg-shaped hyper-reflective structures measuring between 10 and 30 μm with sometimes a double-wall appearance (Fig. 4.2d, e). IVCM may also be able to provide images of trophozoites in AK; however, their exact morphology remains undetermined (Fig. 4.2f). IVCM also showed irregularly thickened nerves evocative of radial keratoneuritis in some cases, modifications of the corneal stroma with hypo-reflective cavities, extensive stromal scarring and stromal edema, infiltration by hyper-reflective inflammatory cells, and highly reflective activated keratocytes.

Numerous publications have supported the use of IVCM as a noninvasive tool to monitor progression and the response to antimicrobial treatment, particularly in cases of *Acanthamoeba* or fungal corneal infections [2], which may be helpful to differentiate between the progression of infection and the toxic effects of therapy.

Corneal Dystrophies

IVCM has been used, since the last 15 years, to examine the cornea in a wide range of corneal dystrophies [5]. This in vivo histological-like approach of corneal dystrophies

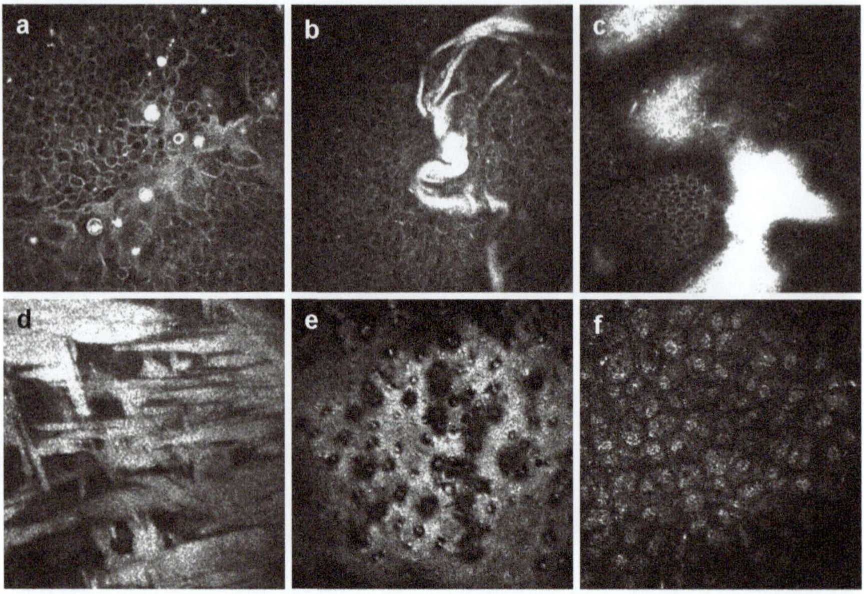

Fig. 4.3 In vivo confocal microscopy (IVCM) images (400×400 μm, Heidelberg Retina Tomograph – Rostock Cornea Module (HRT-RCM)) of corneal dystrophies. Microcysts in the basal epithelial layer in Meesman's corneal dystrophy (**a**). Aberrant thickened basement membrane penetrating into the epithelium in epithelial basement membrane dystrophy (EBMD) (**b**). Granular hyper-reflective material within the basal epithelium and the Bowman's layer in Reis-Bucklers dystrophy (**c**). Large extracellular crystalline deposits in the stroma in Schnyder crystalline dystrophy (**d**). Guttae at the level of the endothelium in Fuchs' endothelial dystrophy (**e**). Epithelioid cells with irregular size and shape, indistinct borders, and hyper-reflective nuclei in iridocorneal endothelial syndrome (**f**)

may assist clinicians not only in the diagnosis but also in their treatment decision. The list of epithelial and stromal dystrophies studied with IVCM includes epithelial basement membrane (EBMD), Meesman's, Reis-Bücklers, Thiel-Behnke, central mosaic, central cloudy dystrophy of François, lattice, granular, Avellino (or granular-lattice), macular central dystrophy, and Schnyder dystrophies.

In Meesman's corneal dystrophy, IVCM showed hypo-reflective areas corresponding to microcysts in the basal epithelial layer associated with large elongated epithelial clefts and round hyper-reflective structures probably corresponding to intracellular material (Fig. 4.3a) [6].

In EBMD patients, IVCM showed the presence of abnormal hyper-reflective linear structures or curved ridges within the intermediate and basal cell layers corresponding to an aberrant thickened basement membrane penetrating into the epithelium. This abnormal basement membrane was also associated with epithelial cell abnormalities and microcysts (Fig. 4.3b) [7].

In Bowman's layer dystrophies, IVCM demonstrated an abnormal reflective tissue replacing the normal bowman's layer. Moreover, IVCM may be able to identify and to differentiate in vivo Thiel-Behnke and Reis-Bucklers corneal dystrophies [8].

In Reis-Bucklers dystrophy, a small granular hyper-reflective material was observed within the basal epithelium and the Bowman's layer (Fig. 4.3c). Distinctively, in Thiel-Behnke dystrophy, the deposits showed homogeneous reflectivity with round edges and dark shadows.

In Schnyder dystrophy, IVCM showed large extracellular crystalline deposits and a highly reflective extracellular matrix modify the corneal architecture with disruption of subepithelial nerve plexus (Fig. 4.3d).

In Fuchs' endothelial dystrophy, using IVCM, guttae appear as round hypo-reflective structures with sometimes a central reflective material at the level of the endothelium. These images are associated with a cellular polymegethism, a pleomorphism, and a decrease in endothelial cell density as evaluated quantitatively with IVCM (Fig. 4.3e). IVCM images of posterior polymorphous dystrophy showed curvilinear and vesicular abnormalities with focal clusters of dark and bright bodies associated with streaks and craters at the level of the Descemet membrane. In iridocorneal endothelial syndrome (ICE syndrome), IVCM images of the endothelium show epithelioid cells with irregular size and shape, indistinct borders, and hyper-reflective nuclei (Fig. 4.3f).

Refractive Surgery

Refractive surgery is one of the areas where IVCM may be the most useful as it can be used to characterize in vivo cellular changes associated with the wound healing response, to evaluate different techniques, or to assess complications [9, 10]. The appearance of the epithelium, the corneal stroma, the interface, the keratocytes or the corneal nerves can be observed and analyzed over time and monitored noninvasively at high resolution.

After PRK, IVCM shows the regeneration of the epithelium that covers the wound. In the anterior stroma, keratocytes become hyper-reflective with visible cellular processes and with an increased density during the early post operative period (Fig. 4.4a). Using IVCM, it has been observed that activated keratocytes were responsible for the clinically visible haze and interestingly, this corneal reaction could be evaluated quantitatively and objectively with this imaging technique [9]. Corneal nerves regeneration after PRK has also been evaluated using IVCM.

Numerous studies on LASIK have been conducted with IVCM. LASIK corneas exhibit microfolds at the level of Bowman's layer appearing as long dark lines with varying thickness and length, often vertically oriented. Observation of the flap interface commonly demonstrates highly reflective particles of variable dimensions (Fig. 4.4b). However, the exact origin of these particles remains undetermined [11]. The density of keratocytes could be measured precisely with a decrease number of keratocytes in the initial wound healing phase on both sides of the cut, in the flap and in the anterior cornea bed. A progressive loss of keratocytes in these areas was also observed 3 years after LASIK [12]. In the meantime other keratocytes below and above the flap show signs of activation with reflective nuclei and visible cytoplasmic processes [11]. IVCM studies of corneal nerves after LASIK have shown that in the sub-basal and stromal flap regions, the number of nerve fiber bundles

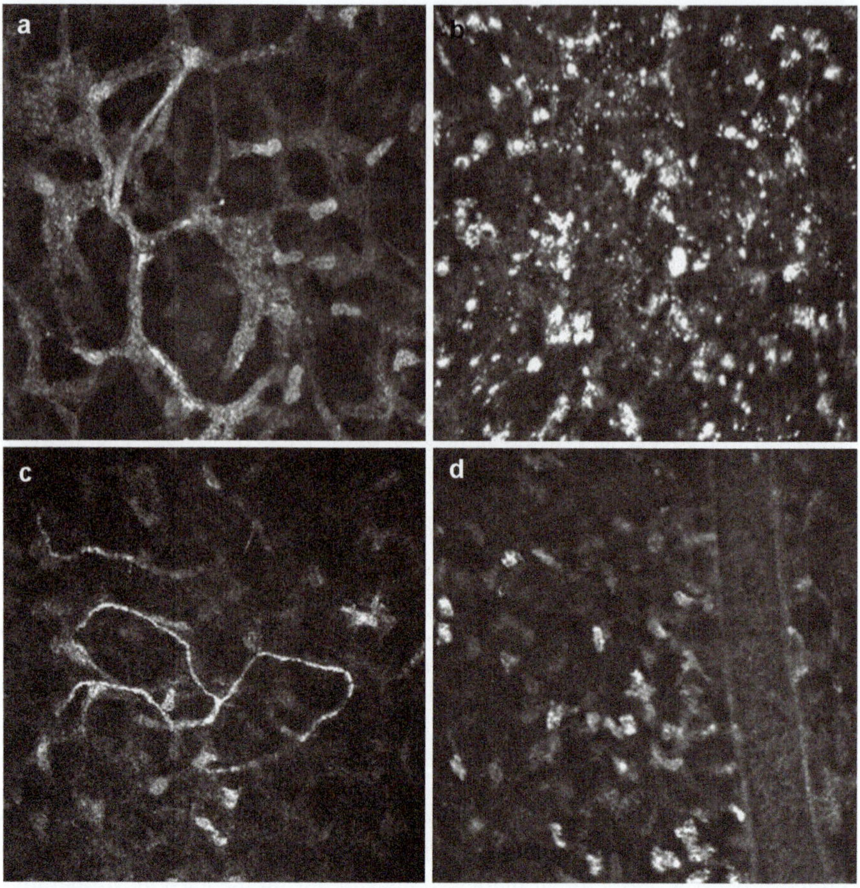

Fig. 4.4 In vivo confocal microscopy (IVCM) images (400×400 μm, Heidelberg Retina Tomograph – Rostock Cornea Module (HRT-RCM)) of the cornea after refractive surgery. Activated keratocytes are hyper-reflective with visible cellular processes (**a**). Flap interface with highly reflective particles of variable dimensions (**b**). Abnormal corneal nerves (**c**). Flap margin after IntraLase® flap creation (**d**)

decreased by more than 90% 1 week after LASIK. Sub-basal and stromal flap nerve fiber bundles gradually increased from month 3 up to 1 year postoperatively, but regeneration appears to remain incomplete for as long as 3 years postoperatively (Fig. 4.4c) [13].

Complications of refractive surgery have also been studied with IVCM [9]. In cases of corneal infiltrate, IVCM could help to differentiate diffuse lamellar keratitis (DLK) with infiltration of cells considered most likely to be mononuclear cells and granulocytes into the interface flap, from infectious keratitis. Finally, IVCM is interesting to characterize and compare the wound healing response and the corneal changes in novel techniques or devices used for refractive surgery (Fig. 4.4) [11].

Corneal Surgery

IVCM was used in numerous studies to evaluate corneal wound healing following penetrating or lamellar keratoplasty, corneal cross-linking, or amniotic membrane transplantation.

As all corneal cells could be evaluated with IVCM, this technique is not only helpful for the preoperative evaluation of the cornea, but also for the follow-up of corneal changes after penetrating keratoplasty. Significant reductions in epithelial cell, keratocyte, nerve and endothelial cell densities were demonstrated with IVCM [14]. Interestingly, IVCM images of corneal allograft rejections revealed focal accumulations of hyper-reflective dendritic-like cells, presumably Langerhans cells, at the level of the basal epithelium and Bowman's membrane associated with altered keratocytes and may be an interesting tool to aid in the diagnosis of early rejection [15].

More recently, IVCM has also been used to analyze the interface of deep lamellar keratoplasty, to compare different surgical techniques, and to measure the interface depth after anterior lamellar keratoplasty, or to evaluate the cornea after Descemet stripping endothelial keratoplasty (DSAEK) or Descemet stripping with automated endothelial keratoplasty (DSAEK).

IVCM can show directly photopolymerization effects and possible complications of corneal cross-linking. After the procedure, rarefaction of keratocytes in the anterior and intermediate stroma, and a stromal edema have been observed without endothelial cell damage. After 6 months, keratocyte population was normal and associated with an increased density of stromal fibers [16].

The observation of the morphology of transplanted amniotic membrane as well as its degradation is also possible with IVCM. The amniotic membrane stroma appears as a superficial dense fibrous layer and a deeper network of loosely arranged fibers

Other Clinical Applications

The long-term success of glaucoma filtering surgery is mainly dependent on the development of a functioning filtering bleb. IVCM allows the visualization of epithelial microcysts, sub-epithelial connective tissue, blood vessels, and inflammatory cells within conjunctival bleb tissues (Fig. 4.5a, b) [17]. Clinicians, with images at a cellular level, would be able to better predict the outcome of these blebs and eventually to provide specific treatments in order to enhance success rates of their surgical procedures.

Contact lens-induced corneal changes have been also described with IVCM. This technique was used to compare various types of lens material and for the diagnosis of corneal complications.

Numerous corneal changes associated with a variety of systemic and/or ocular diseases were described using IVCM: diabetes, Fabry's disease, nephropathic cystinosis (Fig. 4.5c), Marfan syndrome, keratoconus, keratopathy associated with the use of systemic medications such as Amiodarone (Fig. 4.5d) or chloroquine, dry eye, atopic keratoconjunctivitis, or uveitis.

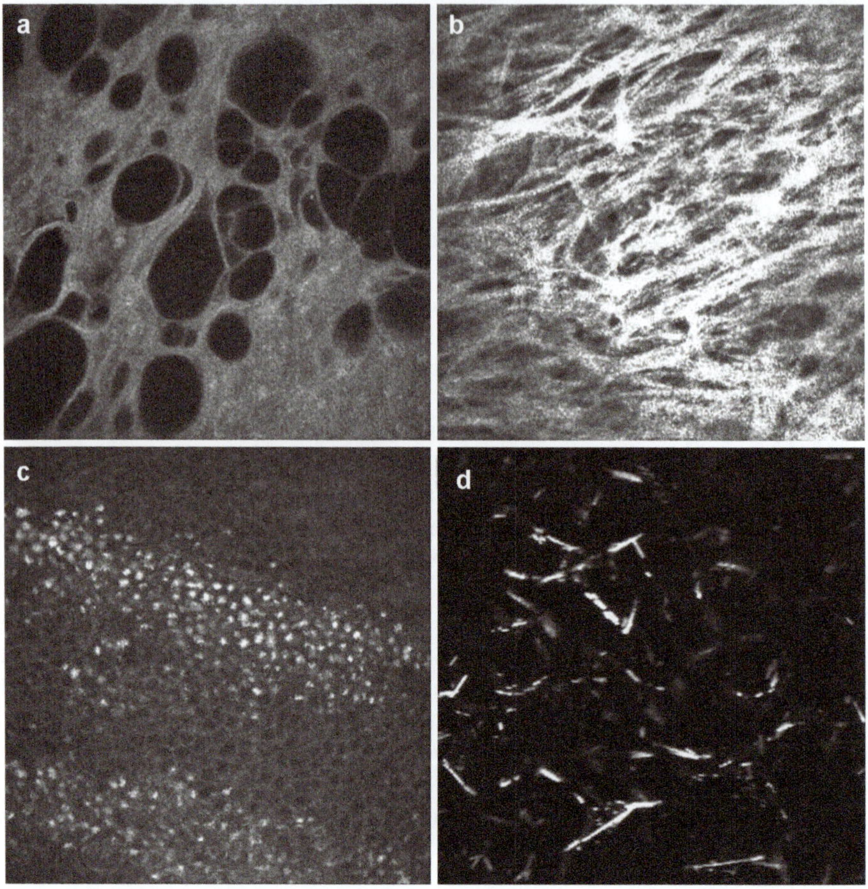

Fig. 4.5 In vivo confocal microscopy (IVCM) images (400×400 μm, Heidelberg Retina Tomograph – Rostock Cornea Module (HRT-RCM)). Numerous microcysts within the epithelium in a functioning filtering bleb (**a**). A dense connective tissue in a non-functioning bleb (**b**). Amiodarone corneal epithelium deposits (**c**). Crystal deposits in the corneal epithelium in the stroma in nephropathic cystinosis (**d**)

Limitations of IVCM

A high degree of compliance is needed to obtain high-resolution images and to carry out a dynamic examination. IVCM remains a contact diagnostic tool and in highly sensitive eyes, the IVCM analysis may cause ocular discomfort and thus increase eye movements that may blur the images.

IVCM, to be really useful, must be performed and interpreted by an experienced operator. As many structures are untypical, images should be interpreted carefully. Because IVCM's field of view is small, the operator has to move the objective over the ocular surface tissues. Similarly, when IVCM is used to follow changes in repeated examinations, one of the major limitations is the difficulty of imaging the same area over time.

Finally, the current resolution and the absence of staining limit IVCM to morphological analyses. Further developments in microscope objectives and image processing will certainly increase the resolution for a more accurate morphological analysis. IVCM of the future should also include the use of staining procedures administered by instillation to facilitate image interpretation and the diagnostic ability of IVCM.

Anterior Segment Ocular Coherence Tomography (OCT)

Analysis of the anterior segment structures is an integral part of ophthalmologic investigations and many clinical situations require a precise assessment not only of the spatial relationships but also of the dimensions of the structures making up this segment of the eye. In everyday clinical practice, corneal imaging is usually carried out with the slit lamp. However, this technique does not provide the means for objective quantitative assessment. New imaging techniques such as anterior segment OCT have thus been developed to overcome these problems.

Principles of Anterior Segment Optical Coherence Tomography (AS-OCT)

Optical coherence tomography is a noninvasive technique which uses a low coherence interferometry principle cross sections of tissue structures in vivo. The technique measures the delay and intensity of the light reflected from the structure being analyzed and compares it with the light reflected by a reference mirror, and the combination of these two signals results in a phenomenon termed interference. The signal intensity depends on the optical properties of the tissues, and the device uses this record to construct a sagittal cross section of the structure being examined. In fact, the operating principle behind OCT is similar to that of the ultrasound scan except that a light is used instead of ultrasound.

Since the speed of light is a million times faster than that of ultrasound, this type of imaging allows longitudinal resolution levels of the order of a few microns to be achieved. Marketed for the first time in 1995 by Carl Zeiss Meditec (Dublin, USA), OCT has until now mostly been used in ophthalmology to produce images of the posterior segment of the eye. The first optical coherence images of the anterior segment were made in 1994 using an OCT with a wavelength of 820 nm designed for examination of the posterior segment. This new imaging technique was then used to assess anatomical changes during refractive surgery and, adapted for use with the slit lamp, for routine clinical examination of the anterior segment. However, the anterior segment images obtained with this system were not always very good in quality. This is because the time taken for image acquisition was between 1 and 5 s, meaning that distortion due to micro-movements of the eye could not be avoided. In addition, the image calculation algorithm designed for the (concave) retina could produce distortions in the images of the (convex) cornea and anterior segment. Finally, the wavelength of 820 nm gave only limited penetration of the signal through the sclera, limbus or iris, making it impossible to view more posterior structures.

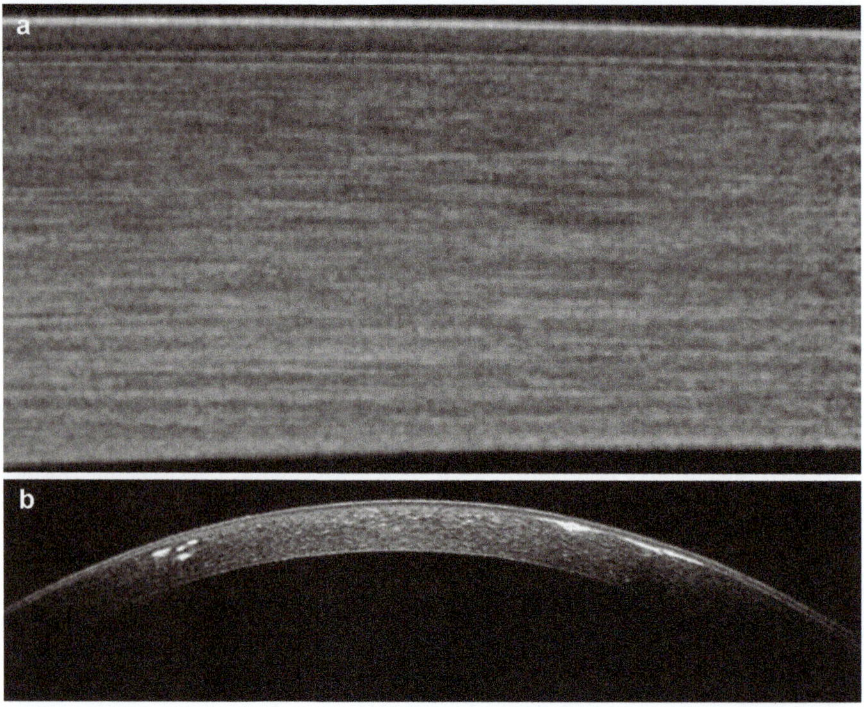

Fig. 4.6 Spectral domain anterior segment ocular coherence tomography (SD-OCT) images of a normal cornea (**a**) and in a case of Avellino corneal dystrophy (**b**)

It was only in 2001 that a high-speed OCT (8 images per second) became available using a wavelength of 1,310 nm allowing optimum visualization of the anterior segment. This wavelength gives better penetration through light-retaining tissues such as the sclera or limbus, making it possible to analyze the iridocorneal angle. Since then, new spectral-domain OCTs have been commercially available for the analysis of the anterior segment and the cornea in particular. As a new imaging technique providing the means of obtaining cross sections of the anterior segment in vivo, anterior segment OCT (AS-OCT) has already found many applications.

Clinical Applications

Corneal Thickness Assessment

Naturally, biometric assessment of the anterior segment has drawn great benefit from this reproducible and totally noninvasive technique. New AS-OCT devices are able to measure the whole corneal thickness as well as the thickness of each corneal layer from the epithelium to the endothelium, allowing to determine the exact depth of corneal deposits susceptible to benefit from phototherapeutic keratectomy (Fig. 4.6). AS-OCT-measured corneal pachymetry is reliable, reproducible, and

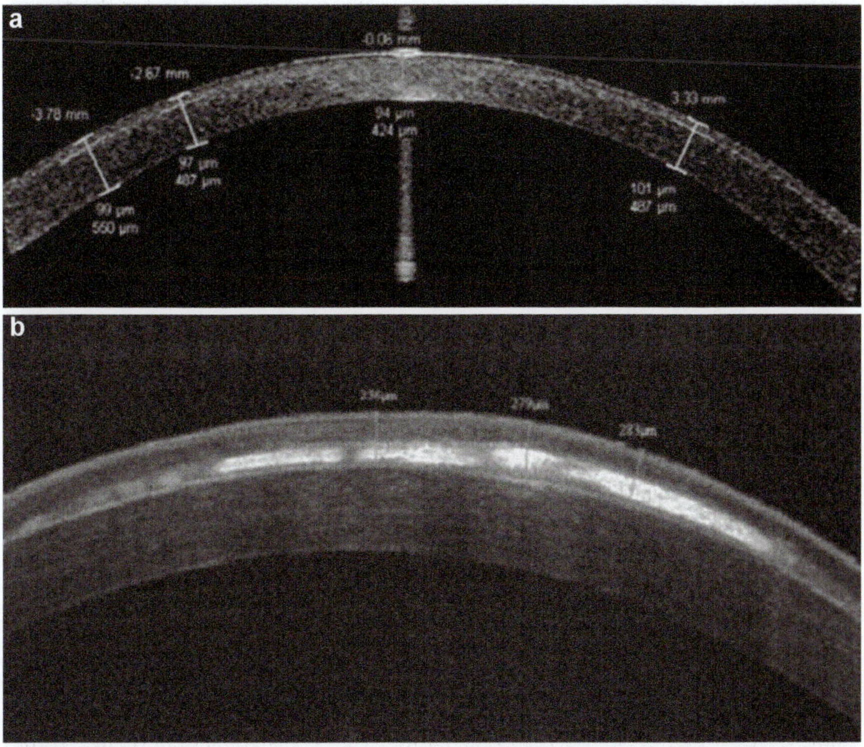

Fig. 4.7 Anterior segment ocular coherence tomography (AS-OCT, Visante OCT®) images. Evaluation of an Intralase® flap after LASIK (**a**). Epithelial ingrowth after LASIK (**b**), the epithelial ingrowth appears as hyper-reflective deposits within the flap with an increased flap thickness

closely correlated with ultrasound pachymetry, especially using Stratus or Fourier-domain OCTs [18, 19]. Three-dimensional mapping of the epithelial thickness may also be greatly improved, even though these new data have still to be validated.

Refractive Surgery

Corneal refractive surgery, including surface ablation, laser in situ keratomileusis, femtosecond laser-assisted flaps (Fig. 4.7a, b) and intracorneal rings (Fig. 4.8), induces deep changes in corneal morphology and optical properties along with cell structure remodeling. Great improvements in corneal imaging allow today microscopic in vivo follow-up of mechanisms involved in corneal wound healing, becoming helpful tools for optimizing our therapeutic decision as well as our surgical procedure.

Preoperatively, high-resolution AS-OCTs, that is, Stratus and Fourier-domain OCTs allow precise measurement of corneal thickness, intracorneal scar localization and volume, or previous LASIK interface depth using qualitative imaging but also quantitative A-mode. Moreover, corneal hydration as well as corneal refractive index can nowadays be assessed thanks to new interferometry-based imaging

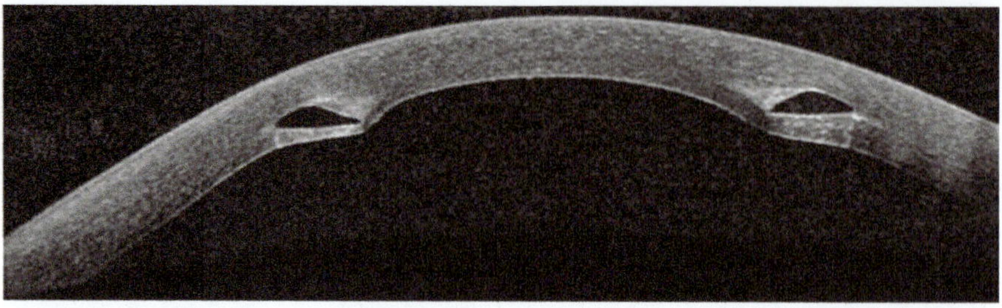

Fig. 4.8 Spectral domain anterior segment ocular coherence tomography (SD-OCT, Spectralis®) image of corneal rings for keratoconus

procedures [20]. After corneal refractive photoablation, wound healing can be followed in vivo with three-dimensional mapping of epithelial or entire corneal thickness using high-resolution AS-OCT [21]. LASIK flaps can be precisely imaged from the center to the edges, and light diffraction at the interface can be measured in order to investigate its influence on contrast perception. Indeed, femtosecond LASER-assisted LASIK has been demonstrated to perform more precise and homogenous flap cutting thanks to AS-OCT imaging [22]. Moreover, measuring changes in corneal curvature and refractive index allows today a better understanding of the relation between corneal ablation and refractive changes, becoming an essential tool before secondary corneal/intraocular surgery.

Complicated evolution of corneal remodeling and/or refraction pattern after corneal surgery can be analyzed using high-resolution AS-OCT to better identify causal mechanisms, from slight epithelial remodeling to true ectasia. Flap interface deposits or micro-folds can be easily characterized combining AS-OCT and confocal microscopy in order to better define the therapeutic strategy. Indeed, AS-OCT is able to show undiagnosed micro-folds which might be responsible for postoperative visual impairments [23]. Secondary structural pathologies including basal membrane dystrophy and Salzmann's-like nodular degeneration can be complementarily diagnosed using high-resolution AS-OCT.

Additionally, in the field of phakic implants, the work by G. Baikoff has clearly demonstrated the advantages of AS-OCT for preoperative assessment of the exact dimensions of the anterior chamber prior to implantation, and for the analysis and follow-up of relationships between the cornea, the phakic IOL, and the lens after implantation (Fig. 4.9a, b) [24].

Corneal Grafts

Imaging of the ocular anterior structures is one of the key points in the analysis and follow-up of corneal grafts. AS-OCT provides today useful qualitative and quantitative data, especially by imaging corneal architecture in new procedures for corneal graft such as deep anterior lamellar keratoplasty and endothelial graft. Moreover, AS-OCT contributes to the diagnosis of postoperative complications by investigating the graft neighboring and imaging the other anterior structures, offering special usefulness when pathological corneal changes make standard clinical examination difficult.

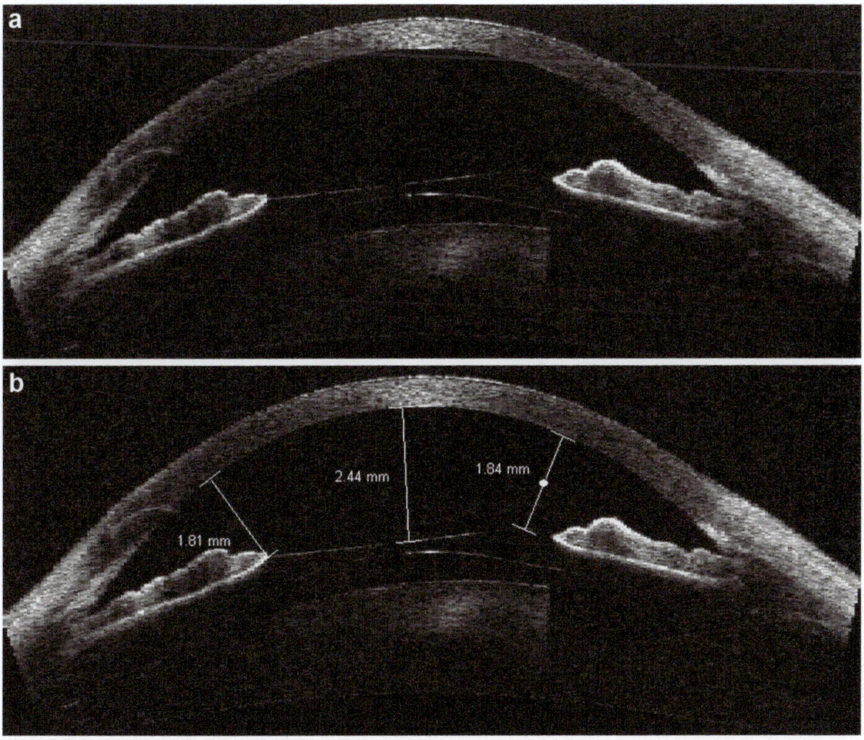

Fig. 4.9 Anterior segment ocular coherence tomography (AS-OCT, Visante OCT®) image of a phakic intraocular lens (**a**) with quantitative measures (**b**)

After penetrating keratoplasty, AS-OCT allows to analyze the entire graft position as well as its macroscopic features such as thickness and curvature (Fig. 4.10a). Since laser-assisted penetrating keratoplasty was developed, AS-OCT has become a useful tool to assess the interface between the graft and the cornea, contributing to the improvement of surgical techniques. Moreover, long-term complications such as descemet membrane rupture or secondary glaucoma can be better diagnosed using AS-OCT even when important edema exists. In new graft procedures, AS-OCT helps to analyze preoperatively the corneal disease along with the anterior segment dimensions in order to better define the right procedure.

Postoperative management of new developments in endothelial grafts, that is, Descemet stripping automated endothelial keratoplasty (DSAEK) has been dramatically improved thanks to AS-OCT (Fig. 4.10b) by following the corneal thickness related to endothelial function [25] as well as by diagnosing early and late complications including Descemet detachment or late pupillary blockade due to iris-graft synechiae. Other unexpected complications such as epithelial ingrowth in the interface can be imaged using AS-OCT.

Last, AS-OCT can substitute for clinical examination after amniotic membrane graft by following in vivo the corneal wound healing above the graft as well as the amniotic membrane integration into the superficial cornea.

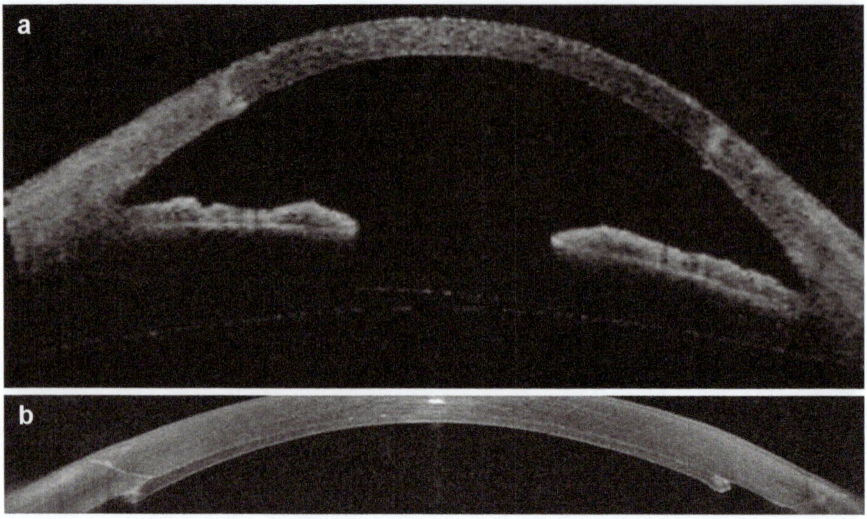

Fig. 4.10 Anterior segment ocular coherence tomography (AS-OCT, Visante OCT®) image after penetrating keratoplasty showing a perfect interface between the cornea and the corneal graft (**a**). Spectral domain anterior segment ocular coherence tomography (SD-OCT, Spectralis®) image of a Descemet stripping automated endothelial keratoplasty (DSAEK) (**b**)

Limitations

AS-OCT provides in vivo imaging of the entire cornea architecture. Developments of new systems based on different wavelengths and on better signal transduction and computerization have improved the spatial resolution as well as deep structure analyses. However, AS-OCT imaging is not able to reach the micrometric precision of IVCM yet. Even if it is a non-contact technique, it requires experienced operator to perform right acquisition and accurate image analysis. Reliability of the pachymetric measurements should be better assessed and improved in order to reach the gold standard that is still ultrasound measurement. Until today, AS-OCT offers axial imaging only, but new experimental devices should be able to perform plano imaging in the future.

Conclusion

IVCM and AS-OCT are noninvasive imaging techniques that provide high-resolution images of the cornea, and numerous clinical applications have been demonstrated for both instruments. IVCM, by providing in vivo histological like images of the cornea, has been largely used in infectious keratitis, corneal dystrophies, and refractive surgery. AS-OCT by offering noninvasive cross sections of the anterior segment has demonstrated its usefulness in refractive and anterior segment surgery, as well as in corneal graft. Hence IVCM and AS-OCT offer complementary qualitative and quantitative data about the corneal structure, from micrometric cell imaging to 3D mapping of the corneal architecture. The future of these techniques will be a better resolution but also the development of vital dyes, 3D and 2D image reconstruction softwares, and perhaps a combination of both techniques providing an in vivo noninvasive reconstruction at the cellular level of corneal and anterior segment structures.

Conflict of Interest The authors have no proprietary or commercial interest in any product or concept discussed in this article.

References

1. Zhivov A, Stachs O, Kraak R et al (2006) In vivo confocal microscopy of the ocular surface. Ocul Surf 4(2):81–93
2. Labbe A, Khammari C, Dupas B et al (2009) Contribution of in vivo confocal microscopy to the diagnosis and management of infectious keratitis. Ocul Surf 7(1):41–52
3. Brasnu E, Bourcier T, Dupas B et al (2007) In vivo confocal microscopy in fungal keratitis. Br J Ophthalmol 91(5):588–591
4. Kaufman SC, Musch DC, Belin MW et al (2004) Confocal microscopy: a report by the American Academy of Ophthalmology. Ophthalmology 111(2):396–406
5. Niederer RL, McGhee CN (2010) Clinical in vivo confocal microscopy of the human cornea in health and disease. Prog Retin Eye Res 29(1):30–58
6. Patel DV, Grupcheva CN, McGhee CN (2005) Imaging the microstructural abnormalities of meesmann corneal dystrophy by in vivo confocal microscopy. Cornea 24(6):669–673
7. Labbe A, Nicola RD, Dupas B et al (2006) Epithelial basement membrane dystrophy: evaluation with the HRT II Rostock Cornea Module. Ophthalmology 113(8):1301–1308
8. Kobayashi A, Sugiyama K (2007) In vivo laser confocal microscopy findings for Bowman's layer dystrophies (Thiel-Behnke and Reis-Bucklers corneal dystrophies). Ophthalmology 114(1):69–75
9. Kaufman SC, Kaufman HE (2006) How has confocal microscopy helped us in refractive surgery? Curr Opin Ophthalmol 17(4):380–388
10. Jalbert I, Stapleton F, Papas E et al (2003) In vivo confocal microscopy of the human cornea. Br J Ophthalmol 87(2):225–236
11. Sonigo B, Iordanidou V, Chong-Sit D et al (2006) In vivo corneal confocal microscopy comparison of intralase femtosecond laser and mechanical microkeratome for laser in situ keratomileusis. Invest Ophthalmol Vis Sci 47(7):2803–2811
12. Erie JC, Nau CB, McLaren JW et al (2004) Long-term keratocyte deficits in the corneal stroma after LASIK. Ophthalmology 111(7):1356–1361
13. Calvillo MP, McLaren JW, Hodge DO, Bourne WM (2004) Corneal reinnervation after LASIK: prospective 3-year longitudinal study. Invest Ophthalmol Vis Sci 45(11):3991–3996
14. Niederer RL, Perumal D, Sherwin T, McGhee CN (2007) Corneal innervation and cellular changes after corneal transplantation: an in vivo confocal microscopy study. Invest Ophthalmol Vis Sci 48(2):621–626
15. Niederer RL, Sherwin T, McGhee CN (2007) In vivo confocal microscopy of subepithelial infiltrates in human corneal transplant rejection. Cornea 26(4):501–504
16. Mazzotta C, Balestrazzi A, Traversi C et al (2007) Treatment of progressive keratoconus by riboflavin-UVA-induced cross-linking of corneal collagen: ultrastructural analysis by Heidelberg Retinal Tomograph II in vivo confocal microscopy in humans. Cornea 26(4):390–397
17. Labbe A, Dupas B, Hamard P, Baudouin C (2005) In vivo confocal microscopy study of blebs after filtering surgery. Ophthalmology 112(11):1979

18. Prakash G, Agarwal A, Jacob S (2009) Comparison of Fourier-domain and time-domain optical coherence tomography for assessment of corneal thickness and intersession repeatability. Am J Ophthalmol 148(2):282–90.e2
19. Simpson T, Fonn D (2008) Optical coherence tomography of the anterior segment. Ocul Surf 6(3):117–127
20. Knuttel A, Bonev S, Knaak W (2004) New method for evaluation of in vivo scattering and refractive index properties obtained with optical coherence tomography. J Biomed Opt 9(2):265–273
21. Li Y, Netto MV, Shekhar R et al (2007) A longitudinal study of LASIK flap and stromal thickness with high-speed optical coherence tomography. Ophthalmology 114(6):1124–1132
22. Stahl JE, Durrie DS, Schwendeman FJ, Boghossian AJ (2007) Anterior segment OCT analysis of thin IntraLase femtosecond flaps. J Refract Surg 23(6):555–558
23. Ustundag C, Bahcecioglu H, Ozdamar A et al (2000) Optical coherence tomography for evaluation of anatomical changes in the cornea after laser in situ keratomileusis. J Cataract Refract Surg 26(10):1458–1462
24. Baikoff G (2006) Anterior segment OCT and phakic intraocular lenses: a perspective. J Cataract Refract Surg 32(11):1827–1835
25. Shih CY, Ritterband DC, Palmiero PM (2009) The use of postoperative slit-lamp optical coherence tomography to predict primary failure in descemet stripping automated endothelial keratoplasty. Am J Ophthalmol 147(5):796–800, e1

Antiangiogenic Treatment Options in the Cornea

5

Claus Cursiefen and Felix Bock

Core Messages

- The cornea uses redundant mechanisms to maintain its evolutionary highly conserved avascular state ("corneal angiogenic privilege").
- Corneal angiogenesis is associated with the most common forms of corneal blindness.
- Corneal angiogenesis is primarily caused by inflammatory diseases of the cornea (e.g., keratitis), corneal hypoxia (contact lens wear), and limbal antiangiogenic barrier defects (most commonly aniridia, chemical burns).
- In corneal inflammation, (hem)angiogenesis (i.e., visible outgrowth of pathologic blood vessels into the cornea) is usually accompanied by lymphangiogenesis (i.e., *invisible* outgrowth of lymphatic vessels).
- Pathologic corneal lymphatic vessels are invisible at the slit-lamp, but can be visualized using specific immunohistochemical markers in explanted vascularized corneas as well as in vivo using HRT confocal microscopy with the cornea module.
- Preexisting blood and even more so lymphatic vessels are strong risk factors for immune rejections after keratoplasty. The same is true for neovascularization developing only after transplantation.

C. Cursiefen, M.D., FEBO (✉) • F. Bock
Department of Ophthalmology, University of Cologne, Joseph-Stelzmann-Strasse 9, Köln D-50924, Germany
e-mail: claus.cursiefen@uk-koeln.de

T. Reinhard, F. Larkin (eds.), *Corneal Disease*,
DOI 10.1007/978-3-642-28747-3_5, © Springer-Verlag Berlin Heidelberg 2013

- Novel antiangiogenic and antilymphangiogenic therapies can improve graft survival both by regression of corneal vessels *prior to* grafting as well as *after* low-risk as well as high-risk keratoplasty by reducing the incidence of immune rejections (novel therapeutic concept).
- Topical and subconjunctival anti-VEGFs are a potent way to treat immature actively outgrowing corneal blood vessels off-label. Safety concerns are development of a neurotrophic keratopathy and inhibition of epithelial and stromal wound healing.
- Targeting Insulin Receptor Substrate –1 is another promising new approach to target both corneal hem-and lymphangiogenesis with an ongoing phase III clinical trial.
- Steroids not only are anti-inflammatory, but also antihem- and antilymphangiogenic. In the transplant context, Prednisolone as the most potent inhibitor of lymphangiogenesis should be used.
- Corneal lymphangiogenesis is not only the prime mediator of corneal graft rejection, but is also involved in the induction of immune-mediated dry eye disease and the induction of ocular surface tumor metastasis.

Introduction

Corneal avascularity is of paramount importance to maintain cornel transparency, the latter being essential for good visual acuity. Therefore, in all higher animals depending on good vision, the cornea normally is devoid of blood and lymphatic vessels ("corneal angiogenic privilege") [1–3]. Nevertheless, several diseases and surgical manipulations can lead to corneal (hem)angiogenesis (i.e., ingrowths of *visible* blood vessels from the limbal vascular arcade into the cornea) and lymphangiogenesis (i.e., ingrowths of *invisible* lymphatic vessels from the limbal vascular arcade into the cornea [1, 2]). Corneal hem- and lymphangiogenesis can cause a significant reduction in visual acuity and blindness as well as render these corneas high-risk in case of a subsequent penetrating or lamellar keratoplasty [1, 2]. In fact, corneal angiogenesis is associated with the most common cause of corneal blindness worldwide (trachoma) as well as the most common form of infectious blindness in western countries (herpetic keratitis [1, 2]). Whereas the animal cornea has been used as in vivo model to study the mechanisms of angiogenesis for decades, the molecular pathways being responsible for maintaining normal avascularity of the human cornea ("angiogenic privilege") are only starting to evolve in recent years [4]. Nonetheless, great progress has been made in recent years to unravel corneal angiogenic and lymphangiogenic privilege [5–8]. Corneal lymphangiogenesis has recently been shown to be of essential importance in the induction of immune responses after corneal transplantation so that novel antihem- and antilymphangiogenic therapies start to emerge as new tools to improve graft survival both in the low-risk as well as the high-risk setting of corneal transplantation [5, 9].

"Angiogenic Privilege of the Cornea" or "How Does the Normal Corneal Maintain Its Avascularity?"

Although the cornea – due to its anatomically exposed position – constantly is in contact with numerous minor inflammatory and thereby angiogenic stimuli, the normal cornea remains avascular [1, 3, 4]. Even after more severe trauma – such as refractive surgery – the cornea in contrast to other tissues – does not respond with angiogenesis. This so-called "angiogenic privilege" [1, 3, 4] is not only essential for good visual acuity but also is responsible for the excellent survival of corneal grafts placed into avascular low-risk recipient beds since in these eyes the graft is physically separated both from the *afferent* (lymphatic) as well as the *efferent* (blood vascular) arm of a so-called *immune reflex arc* leading to immune rejection after keratoplasty [1, 2, 5, 9, 10]. Recent research has shown that the cornea uses several and redundant mechanisms to maintain its avascularity against numerous subthreshold angiogenic stimuli. In fact, several of these mechanisms are very elaborate and examples of how evolutionary important corneal avascularity was. First, the cornea contains numerous endogenous inhibitors of angiogenesis and lymphangiogenesis (such as PEDF, thrombospondins 1 and 2, antiangiogenic matrix cleavage products such as angiostatin and endostatin, IL1RA, etc.) [1, 11]. It seems that these antiangiogenic factors are strategically located at the inner and outer linings of the cornea (Descemet's membrane and epithelial basement membrane) to counteract angiogenic stimuli both from inside (e.g., high concentrations of angiogenic growth factors in the aqueous humor during proliferative diabetic retinopathy) or from outside (e.g., against angiogenic growth factors from the tear film [1, 11]). Animal experiments using mice deficient of one or more antiangiogenic factors (such as thrombospondins 1 and 2) have shown that the corneal angiogenic privilege is *redundantly organized* so that absence of one or two factors does not cause spontaneous ingrowths of limbal blood vessels [3, 4]. This is in contrast to other intraocular tissues such as the iris, where absence of these factors causes increased vascularity [4]. This demonstrates that evolutionary, the cornea has acquired a *robust and redundant antiangiogenic system*, normally maintaining avascularity unless it is overrun by overwhelmingly strong (usually inflammatory/infectious) stimuli for angiogenesis which threaten the integrity of the whole eye or even the whole body [3, 4]. In addition, secondly, the cornea has several receptor decoy mechanisms in place which use "false" receptors to bind and neutralize angiogenic growth factors which would normally cause (lymph) angiogenesis. Examples are the ectopic expression of a VEGF receptor (VEGFR3; Fig. 5.1) on the corneal epithelium, the soluble form of VEGF receptor 1 and 2 as well as Interleukin 1 receptors. A third strategy of the cornea is to block hypoxia-induced forms of angiogenesis by molecularly interfering with hypoxia (HIF)-induced upregulation of angiogenic growth factors in the cornea such as VEGF.

Summary for the Clinician

- Cornea and cartilage are the only avascular tissues of the human body.
- Corneal avascularity is achieved by numerous elaborate and redundant mechanisms in place and actively maintained, e.g. after refractive surgery ("corneal angiogenic privilege").
- Loss of angiogenic privilege, i.e. corneal angiogenesis is associated with and potentially causative for the most common causes of corneal blindness worldwide (trachoma) and the most common form of infectious corneal blindness in industrialized countries (herpetic keratitis)

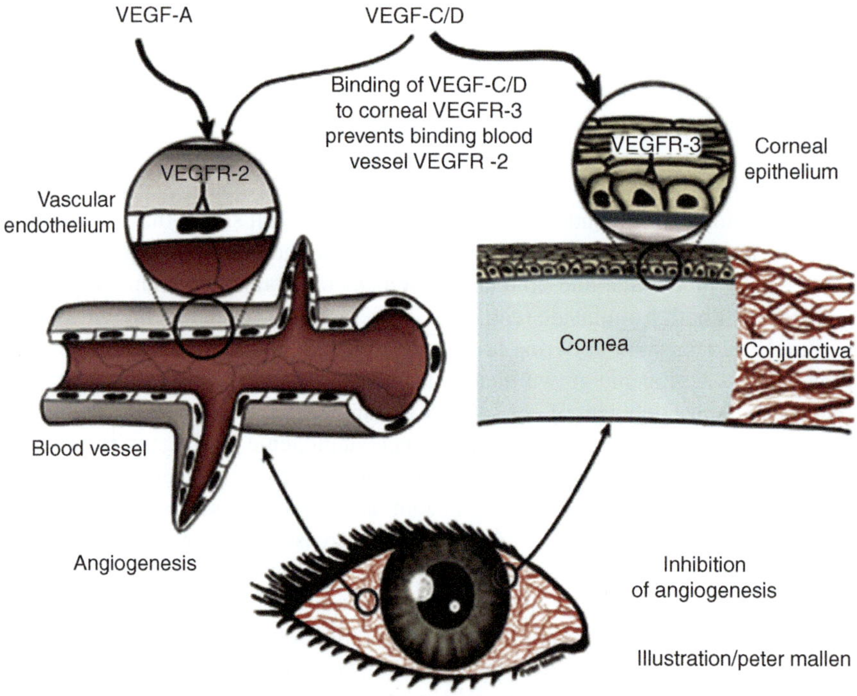

Fig. 5.1 Corneal angiogenic privilege is maintained by multiple and redundant mechanisms. One interesting strategy is the expression of decoy receptors in the cornea, amongst them ectopically expressed VEGF receptor 3 (VEGFR3) in the corneal epithelium. In this ectopic location, the receptor binds and neutralizes angiogenic growth factors such as VEGF-C and -D and prevents their ligation to the normal receptors in adjacent conjunctival vessels, thereby maintaining corneal avascularity (From Ref. [12])

Corneal Hemangiogenesis and Lymphangiogenesis: General Mechanisms and Clinical Features

General Mechanisms

According to FOLKMAN, a balance between angiogenic and antiangiogenic factors in each tissue and situation determines whether angiogenesis occurs or not. If the balance is tipped toward angiogenic growth factors, vessel outgrowth starts ("angiogenic switch"), whereas if inhibitors prevail, angiogenesis is prohibited. Several angiogenic growth factors (primarily growth factors from the VEGF family [VEGF-A, VEGF-C, VEGF-D], FGF, IL1, etc.) as well as inhibitors of angiogenesis have been identified in recent years [13]. Pathologic angiogenesis (to clearly separate this process from *lymph*angiogenesis, we will subsequently refer to it as "*hem*angiogenesis") and lymphangiogenesis into the cornea mainly occur in settings of an inflammatory "insult" to the cornea, corneal hypoxia, or limbal barrier defects, all overriding the *angiogenic privilege* of the cornea, which is actively maintained [3, 4, 12, 14]. Clinical conditions most commonly associated with corneal neovascularization include keratitis (herpetic and bacterial in nature), contact lens wear as well as inherited or acquired limbal deficiency states (primarily chemical burns [3, 4, 12, 14]). In addition, "secondary" corneal angiogenesis can occur after surgical manipulations at the cornea, which primarily involve placement of corneal sutures (e.g., after corneal wound repair, after corneal transplantation, after block excision, etc. [15]). Growth factors of the VEGF family have been identified as key players in both inflammation-driven hem- as well as lymphangiogenesis into the normally avascular cornea [1, 9, 16]. Release of angiogenic growth factors generally is induced primarily by two factors: (a) inflammation and inflammatory cytokines (at the cornea: e.g., keratitis) and (b) hypoxia (at the cornea: e.g., contact lens-induced). The sources for (lymph)angiogenic growth factors within the cornea are multifold, but inflammatory cells and, here especially, macrophages seem to be key players. Early removal of macrophages during an inflammatory insult to the cornea can nearly completely block hem- and lymphangiogenesis in the cornea.

Clinical Consequences of Corneal Hem- and Lymphangiogenesis

Corneal angiogenesis can lead to reduced visual acuity not only by the physical presence of blood vessels itself, but also due to leakage of products from immature corneal blood vessels. This includes corneal edema due to water leakage, corneal lipid keratopathy due to lipid leakage, and intrastromal or subepithelial hemorrhage (e.g., in contact lens patients). In addition, neovascularization can occur into the interface after deep anterior lamellar keratoplasty and cause significant vision loss. Furthermore, as outlined below, corneal angiogenesis impairs the prognosis of corneal grafts placed into vascularized high-risk corneas. In fact, the Collaborative Corneal Transplantation Study [17] (and numerous other clinical as well as experimental studies [2]) revealed preexisting corneal blood vessels as strong(est) risk factor for subsequent immune rejections. In a recent meta-analysis of nearly 25,000 patients having undergone keratoplasty, we showed corneal neovascularization to be a significant risk factor for graft failure and rejection [18]. That risk increased with the number of corneal quadrants being affected by corneal neovascularization.

Summary for the Clinician

- Corneal (lymph)angiogenesis starts when the balance between proangiogenic and antiangiogenic factors in the cornea is shifted toward angiogenic growth factors.
- The most common clinical conditions associated with corneal angiogenesis are corneal inflammation (keratitis), hypoxia (contact lens), and limbal barrier defects (chemical burns).
- Corneal angiogenesis leads to reduced visual acuity by the physical presence of vessels itself, but also by leakage of water, lipids, and erythrocytes.
- Preexisting corneal blood and lymphatic vessels are a strong risk factor for subsequent immune rejections after keratoplasty.

The Importance of Corneal Hem- and Lymphangiogenesis for Immune Reactions After Keratoplasty

Preexisting corneal blood vessels – as mentioned above – have long been identified as strong risk factors for immune rejection after keratoplasty [17]. But, until very recently, the role of the clinically invisible lymphangiogenesis as well as angiogenesis occurring only *after* keratoplasty was unclear [15, 19, 20].

Corneal Hemangiogenesis After Low-Risk Keratoplasty

More than 50 % of patients *after* low-risk keratoplasty (with *pre*operatively avascular corneas), *post*operatively develop corneal angiogenesis within the first year [15]. New vessels are primarily located in the 6 °° and 12 °° position and tend to grow toward the outer suture turning points. In about 10 % of patients, these new vessels actually reach donor tissue. Experiments in the mouse model of low-risk keratoplasty recently have shown that these capillaries are always accompanied by biomicroscopically invisible lymph vessels [7, 9]. Indeed, experiments in the mouse model of low-risk keratoplasty recently identified postkeratoplasty neovascularization as a risk factor for subsequent immune rejections [7, 9]. An antihem- and antilymphangiogenic therapy significantly improved graft survival after low-risk keratoplasty.

Corneal Hemangiogenesis After High-Risk Keratoplasty

Even after high-risk keratoplasty, preexisting blood vessels tend to increase. Only after keratoplasty for herpetic keratitis does removal of the angiogenic stimulus lead to a reduction in corneal angiogenesis. Animal experiments recently clearly demonstrated that even after high-risk keratoplasty there is a significant further increase in both hem- and lymphangiogenesis. In addition, inhibition of these processes even *after* high-risk keratoplasty (in the mouse model) could improve subsequent graft survival. That is true both for "hot" eyes shortly after an inflammation and also for eyes where the inflammation has calmed down and vessels have partly regressed over months ("intermediate risk"). Even in these regressed old high-risk eyes does postkeratoplasty anti-VEGF therapy promote graft survival in the animal model.

Summary for the Clinician

- Corneal angiogenesis postoperatively occurs in about 50 % of patients *after* low-risk keratoplasty in preoperatively avascular recipient beds.
- Animal experiments suggest that hemangiogenesis after keratoplasty is accompanied by clinically invisible lymphangiogenesis.
- Postoperative hem- and lymphangiogenesis have been identified as risk factors for immune rejection after keratoplasty.
- Inhibition of postkeratoplasty angiogenesis and lymphangiogenesis improves graft survival both in the low-risk and high-risk setting (mouse experiments)
- Care should be taken with contact lens-induced corneal angiogenesis in keratoconus patients, since that may compromise the success of a subsequent keratoplasty due to increased risk of immune rejections and may cause interface bleeding after DALK surgery.

Corneal Lymphangiogenesis: Essential for Corneal Graft Rejection

Lymphangiogenesis has recently gained wide interest for its important role in tumor metastasis and induction of alloimmunity after organ transplantation [21]. Whereas it has been known for more than 100 years that the normally avascular cornea can be invaded by blood vessels (hemangiogenesis), it was unclear until very recently whether the normally alymphatic human cornea can be invaded by lymphatic vessels from the lymphatic arcade at the limbus [1, 11]. The main reasons for that unclarity were (1) the fact that lymph vessels – in contrast to erythrocyte-filled blood vessels – are not detectable biomicroscopically using the normal slit-lamp magnification and (2) the lack of specific markers for lymphatic endothelium. The latter has changed in the last 5–10 years with the advent of several specific markers of lymphatic endothelium (such as LYVE-1, Podoplanin, and VEGF receptor 3 [21]). These novel markers enabled for the first time the precise identification of lymphatic vessels in vascularized human corneas [11]. Lymphatic vessels were significantly more common in corneas with a short history of a corneal inflammation (usually keratitis or trauma) and also were significantly more common in heavily vascularized corneas [8]. Thereby, the chance of having both pathological blood as well as clinically invisible lymphatic vessels present is strongly correlated with the degree of corneal angiogenesis, which can be judged by slit-lamp evaluation. Furthermore, recent work shows that it is possible to demonstrate lymphatic vessels in vivo in the cornea using confocal microscopy (HRT II using the Rostock module; see below). Since lymphatic vessels are invisible at slit-lamp magnifications, they might not be as detrimental for corneal transparency as blood vessels are. In fact, animal experiments suggest that the "antilymphangiogenic privilege" of the cornea is not redundantly organized.

Using the mouse model of corneal neovascularization, we recently could demonstrate that after an inflammatory stimulus to the cornea, there is usually parallel and very early (within 48 h) outgrowth of both blood and lymphatic vessels. Both originate from the limbal vascular arcade [7]. The cornea therefore is also an excellent model system to study the mechanisms not only of angiogenesis but also lymphangiogenesis and test pharmacologic compounds for the relative inhibition of both processes in the animal model [14]. Compared to blood vessels, lymphatic vessels tend to regress much quicker and more complete after an inflammatory challenge to the cornea [22]. For example, after a short, 2-week long inflammatory stimulus (corneal sutures), all lymphatic vessels in the mouse cornea are completely regressed after 6 months, whereas blood vessels persist (partly as non-perfused ghost vessels) indefinitely. As outlined below, this supports the clinical practice not to perform penetrating keratoplasties in freshly inflamed eyes, but to wait until inflammation has calmed down to improve graft survival [22]. Lymphangiogenesis is mediated by the VEGF family growth factors VEGF-A, -C and -D as well as by FGF and PDGF [21]. Stimuli for the release of the main lymphangiogenic growth factor VEGF-C are primarily inflammatory in nature, explaining the clinical observation that human corneal lymphangiogenesis is more common shortly after keratitis [8].

The relative higher importance of the afferent *lymphatic* arm of the immune response in dictating the outcome of corneal graft survival has recently been demonstrated by several elegant studies: Indefinite survival of both fully mismatched orthotopic non-high-risk grafts [23] as well as 90 % survival of fully mismatched high-risk corneas [24] in BALB/c-mice was achieved by removal of cervical lymph nodes by cervical lymphadenectomy. Furthermore, pharmacologic strategies inhibiting lymphangiogenesis(and angiogenesis) after low-risk keratoplasty (see Fig. 5.2) and even after high-risk keratoplasty can significantly improve corneal graft survival. In addition, we were recently able to create differentially prevascularized recipient beds in mice. This allowed us to compare the survival rates of grafts placed into completely avascular recipient beds (low-risk setting) as compared to both hem- and lymphvascularized recipient beds (high-risk setting) as compared to only hemvascularized (so-called alymphatic high risk) beds [10] (Fig. 5.2). Interestingly, that showed that there was no difference in survival rates between grafts placed into avascular as compared to grafts placed into only hemvascularized beds. Only if lymphatic vessels were present in addition to blood vessels, the survival rate dropped significantly. That clearly shows that lymphatic vessels are the main "culprit" responsible for the high rate of immune rejections after keratplasty into high-risk recipient beds. All this supports the novel concept that anti*lymph*angiogenic therapies can modulate immune responses after keratoplasty and thereby improve graft survival [10].

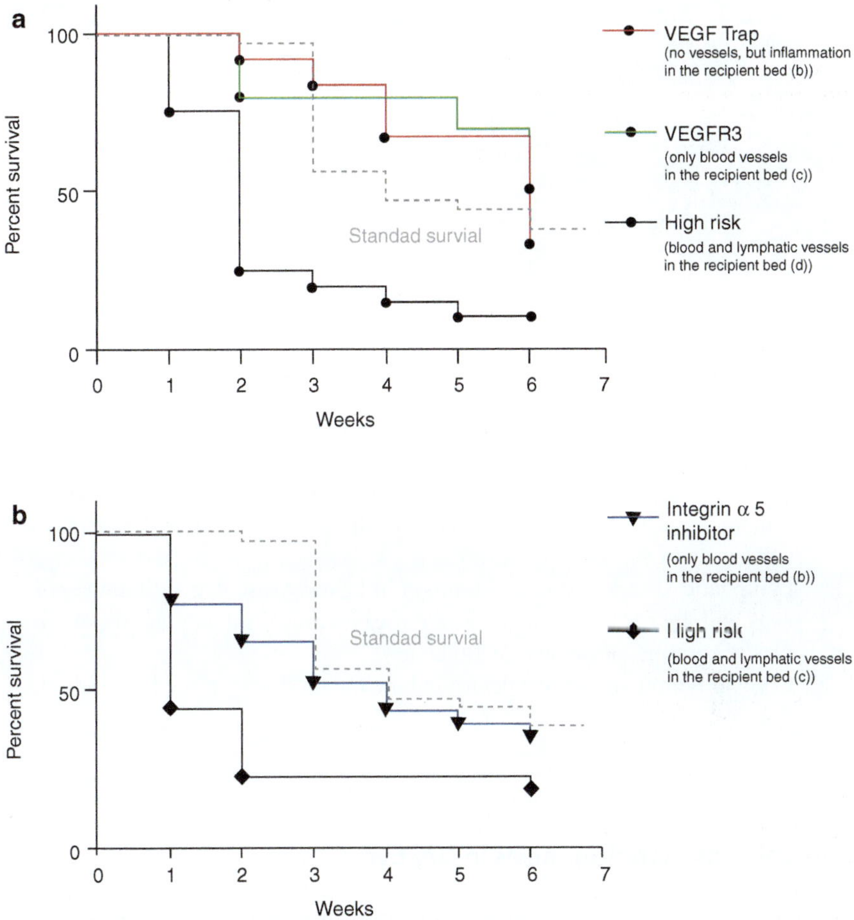

Fig. 5.2 Lymphatic vessels in the recipient bed prior to transplantation determine graft survival: Graft survival was significantly better when transplants were placed into recipient beds lacking lymphatic vessels (*red line*, *green line*, *blue line*) compared to beds with lymphatic vessels being present at the time of transplantation (*black line*) [10]. The presence or absence of blood vessels was not relevant (compare green [d: only blood vessels present] versus red line [c: no vessels at all]). Generation of different transplantation models. Images showing wholemounts of (**c**) avascular high-risk (inflamed, but avascular, recipients), (**d**, **e**) alymphatic high-risk (inflamed and hemvascularized, but no lymphatic vessels), (**f**) high-risk (inflamed and hemvascularized and lymphvascularized) and (**g**) normal risk (avascular) recipient beds as transplantation models

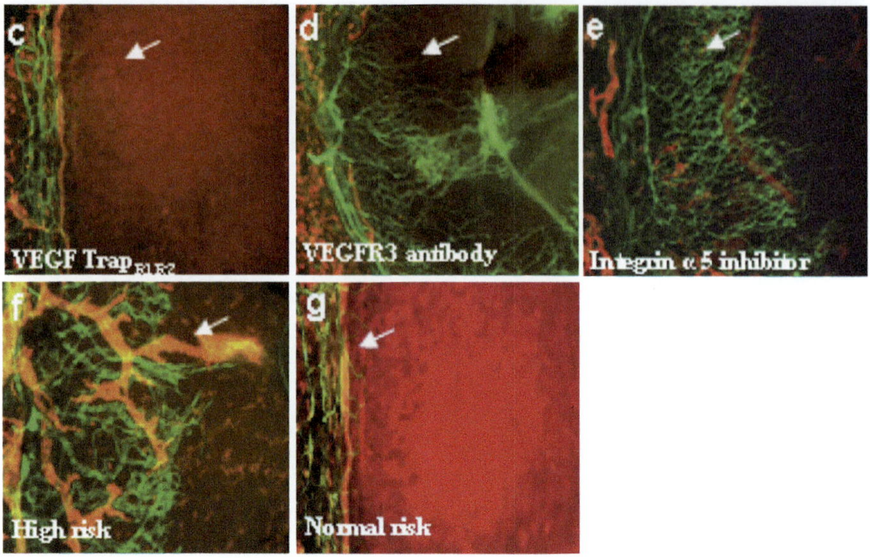

Fig. 5.2 (continued)

> **Summary for the Clinician**
> - During corneal inflammation, there is parallel outgrowth of both blood and lymphatic vessels from the limbus into the cornea (combined *hem*angiogenesis and *lymph*angiogenesis).
> - Lymphatic vessels are more common in heavily vascularized human corneas and are more common shortly after a corneal inflammation (keratoplasty, keratitis, immune rejection, etc.)
> - Corneal lymphatic vessels determine the fate of a graft placed into a high-risk cornea.

Corneal Lymphangiogenesis in Dry Eye

There is preliminary evidence suggesting an involvement of corneal lymphangiogenesis in the disease process of chronic inflammatory dry eye disease. Experimentally, in dry eye models, mild isolated ingrowths of lymphatic vessels into murine corneas can be observed. These lymphatics may act as conduit for the delivery of antigens to regional lymph nodes, thus initiating the chronic "autoimmune" form of dry eye disease. Novel anti(lymph)angiogenic treatment approaches may thus in the future also be part of dry eye treatment.

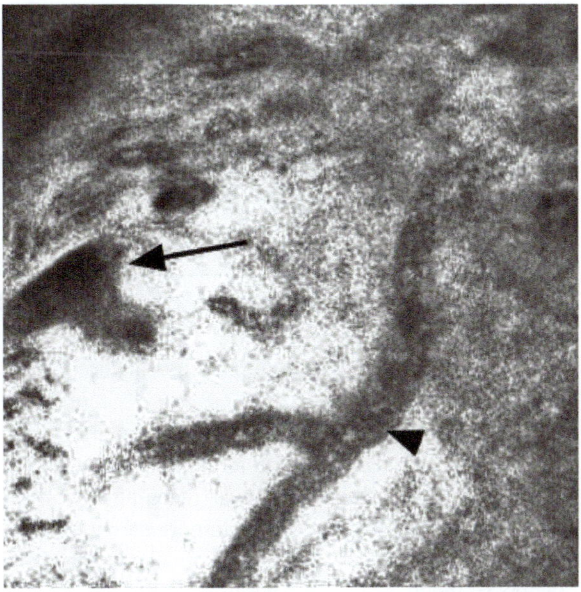

Fig. 5.3 In vivo imaging of corneal lymphatic vessels in a pathologically vascularized murine cornea using in vivo confocal microscopy. The HRT II with the Rostock cornea module shows black, empty appearing, and nearly cell-free lymphatic vessels (*arrow*) next to smaller, erythrocyte-filled blood vessels (*arrowhead*)

Imaging of Corneal Lymphatic Vessels

Lymphatic vessels in the cornea are not visible using slit-lamp magnification. That is due to their lumen being nearly free of cells and their absent basement membrane thus given too low contrast to surrounding extracellular matrix. Nonetheless, in recent years, new technologies have been developed to visualize corneal lymphatics:

(a) *In vivo confocal microscopy using the HRT II and the Rostock cornea module*: Using that approach, we and others were able to visualize lymphatic vessels in rodent corneas. The empty appearing, dark, and cell-free lymphatics could be identified by injection of dyes and subsequent immunohistochemistry. That approach should in the future also be applicable to patients in the clinic (Fig. 5.3).

(b) *In vivo multiphoton imaging*: This even more precise approach allows for unequivocal identification of immunohistochemically labeled lymphatics in the living cornea [35].

Based on the great advances in imaging lymphatics in vivo in animal models, it is likely that in the near future, visualization of lymphatics also in human corneas in the clinic will be possible. That would allow for precise risk assessment prior to keratoplasty by analyzing whether a vascularized high-risk cornea does contain lymphatic vessels in addition or not.

Summary for the Clinician

- Corneal lymphangiogenesis may also be involved in the pathogenesis of chronic dry eye disease.
- Corneal lymphatic vessels can be visualized in vivo in animal corneas using confocal and multiphoton microscopy.

Novel Anti(lymph)Angiogenic Treatment Options at the Cornea

Antiangiogenic therapeutic approaches at the cornea can broadly be divided into two categories:

1. *Angiostatic/antiangiogenic*, i.e. to stop the outgrowths of newly outgrowing immature vessels (classical antiangiogenic approach)
2. *Angioregressive/angioocclusive* (meaning regression of already established mature pathologic vessels, especially important, e.g. in prevascularized high-risk eyes).

Mature, pericyte-covered vessels do not depend on VEGF and other angiogenic growth factors so much, so we need additional physical approaches to close these mature vessels. In contrast for immature vessels, anti-VEGFs are a potent treatment approach.

As outlined above, lymphatic vessels seem to be the prime mediators of corneal graft rejection [10]. That means that in the transplant context, it would most likely be sufficient to block lymphangiogenesis to promote graft survival. Specific inhibitors of lymphangiogenesis are desirable, since these would probably not interfere with corneal wound healing. We and others have recently described several new pharmacological approaches to (relatively) specifically target inflammatory corneal lymphangiogenesis. These approaches include

(a) Blocking peptides against integrins expressed on lymphatic vascular endothelial cells. Blocking peptides against integrin alpha 5, being expressed on lymphatic vascular endothelium in vivo, at certain concentrations relatively specifically block lymph- without affecting hemangiogenesis [25].

(b) Blocking antibodies against the lymphatic vascular endothelial-specific VEGF receptor 3 also have been shown to relatively specifically block inflammatory lymph- without affecting hemangiogenesis [26].

None of these approaches has yet entered clinical trials for use in patients, but they are promising tools for a (relative) specific blockade of lymphangiogenesis in the context of corneal transplantation to promote graft survival in the near future [10].

Current Treatment Options for Immature Corneal (Blood and Lymphatic) Vessels

The drugs available so far to inhibit active corneal (lymph)angiogenesis in the cornea include topical steroids/Cyclosporine A, anti VEGFs (such as Bevacizumab, Ranibizumab, VEGF Trap, and Pegaptanib) as well as GS101/Aganirsen (i.e., strategies targeting IRS-1 signaling). These will be discussed below. Most of these compounds not only inhibit hem- but also lymphangiogenesis.

Steroids

Steroids have long been and still are the mainstay of topical anti-inflammatory treatment in the context of corneal transplantation. Steroids are partly antiangiogenic and as we could recently show also antilymphangiogenic [27]. That effect is mediated not only by inhibiting inflammatory cells influx, but also by direct effects on vascular endothelial cells. The antihem- and antilymphangiogenic potency of steroids significantly varies, with Prednisolone and Dexamethasone being the most potent antilymphangiogenic drugs. That implies that in the transplant context, Prednisolone should be given. Nonetheless, steroids are only partly antiangiogenic and have severe long-term side effects. Therefore, more specific antiangiogenic drugs are needed to achieve more safety and efficacy. In fact, a combined anti-inflammatory and antiangiogenic treatment strategy (e.g., by combining steroids and modern anti-VEGFs) did achieve the best antiangiogenic effect in models of experimental corneal neovascularization (Fig. 5.4).

Anti-VEGFs (Bevazicumab, Ranibuzumab, Pegaptanib, VEGF Trap)

Anti-VEGF pharmacological strategies using Bevacizumab (Avastin®), Ranibizumab (Lucentis®), Pegaptanib (Macugen®), or VEGF Trap® potently inhibit experimental corneal neovascularization. Avastin eye drops, VEGF Trap, and Lucentis eye drops in addition also have been shown to inhibit corneal lymphangiogenesis in animal models [10, 28]. Based on these experimental data, that treatment approach has already been translated into clinical application (Fig. 5.5).

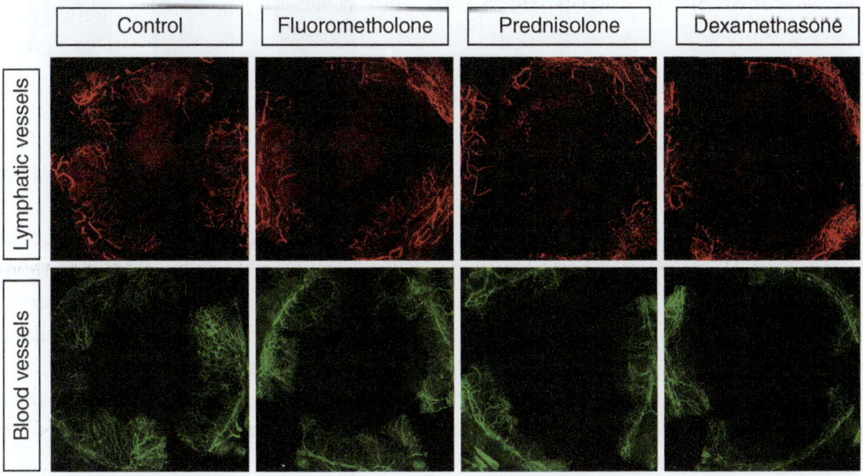

Fig. 5.4 Antihem- and antilymphangiogenic potency of topically applied steroids (From Ref. [27]). There is a significant difference in the antihem- and antilymphangiogenic potency between dexamethasone and prednisolone on one side and fluorometholones on the other side. In the transplant setting therefore, the first two drugs should be applied to effectively block lymphangiogenesis

Fig. 5.4 (continued)

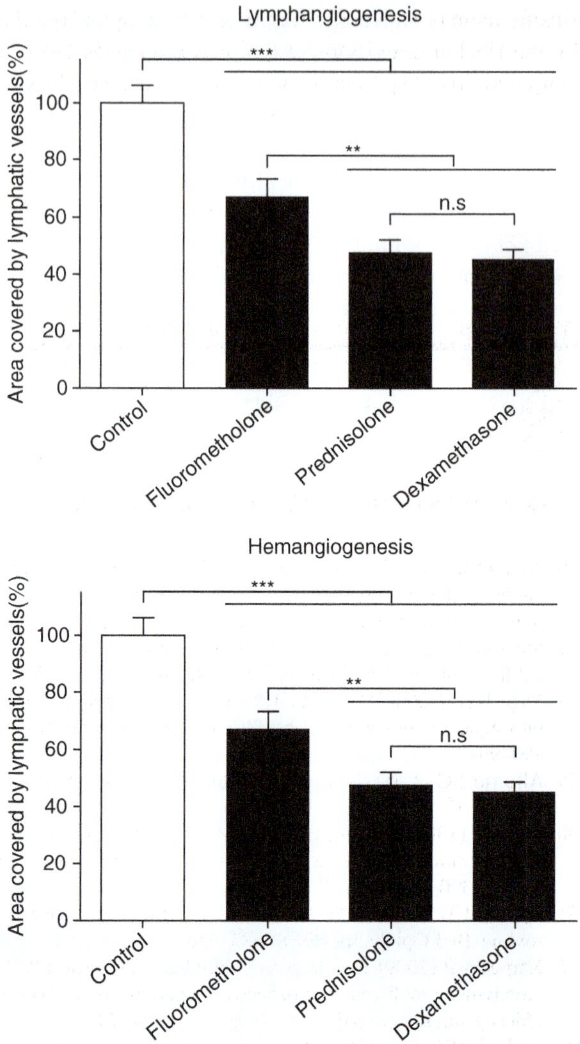

Patients being treated with Avastin eye drops off-label for pathologic corneal neovascularization which were unresponsive to conventional therapy, show a significant but variable response to additional Avastin eye drops when neovascularization was analyzed morphometrically on standardized digitized slit-lamp pictures [29]. We use Avastin in 5 mg/ml dilution 5×/day. Eye drops were well tolerated. Nonetheless, there is concern about wound healing delay and neurotoxic effects by targeting VEGF at the ocular surface. Numerous published case reports, small case series, and also one controlled trial support the concept of Avastin eye drops or subconjunctival applications being relatively effective and relatively safe. Therefore, prospective randomized studies are necessary to define indications, safety, and effectivity of that approach in inhibiting corneal neovascularization.

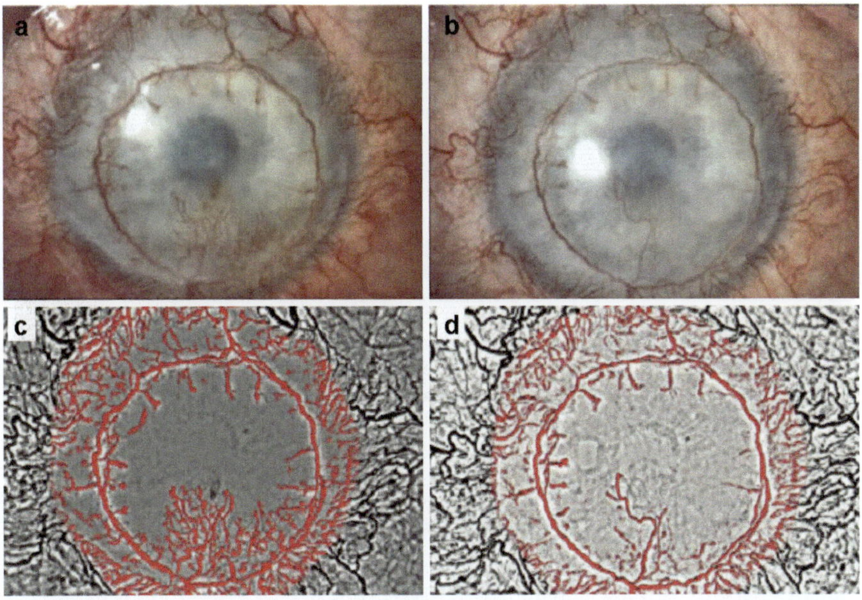

Fig. 5.5 Avastin eye drops significantly inhibit progressive corneal neovascularization (From Ref. [29]). There is a significant decrease of corneal neovessels comparing prior to (**a**) and after additional treatment for 4 weeks with Avastin eye drops (**b**). The respective image analysis is shown in panels (**c**) and (**d**)

For the other two off-label available anti-VEGF agents, there is much less known about their effect on human corneal neovascularization. Initial clinical data suggest that Lucentis eye drops – perhaps because of smaller size and better penetration into the cornea – have an even stronger antiangiogenic effect at the cornea. Preclinical data show both of them being active against corneal neovascularization, with Ranibizumab – as said above – also being active against corneal lymphangiogenesis.

Anti-IRS 1-Strategies (Antisense Oligonucleotides Against IRS 1)

Insulin receptor substrate (IRS) 1 has recently been shown to be a key mediator of inflammatory angiogenesis in several in vivo models. Based on that, an antisense oligonucleotide significantly blocking IRS-1 signaling was developed and tested preclinically and clinically. Phase II trial data from a prospective multicenter randomized European trial recently showed that anti-IRS-1 eye drops (Aganirsen) applied twice daily significantly inhibit progressive corneal neovascularization and are well-tolerated. Animal experimental data show that this compound not only blocks visible hem- but also invisible lymphangiogenesis. Based on the positive phase II data, a randomized phase III trial is currently being conducted in Europe. Anti-IRS-1 treatment strategies may evolve as an effective and safe treatment approach to topically target progressive corneal neovascularization in the future (Fig. 5.6).

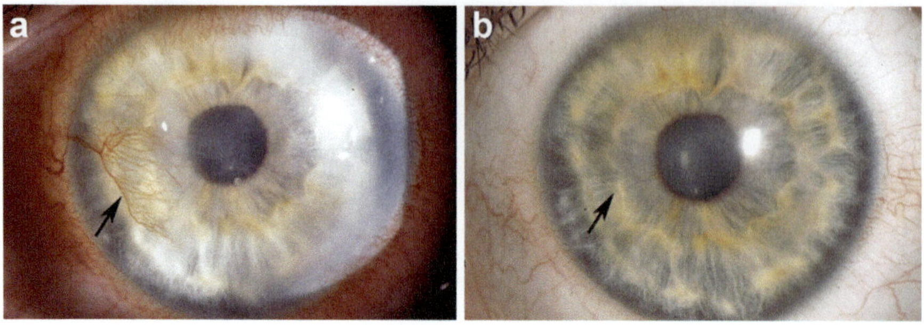

Fig. 5.6 Eye drops with antisense oligonucleotides against IRS-1 given twice daily were shown to significantly inhibit progressive corneal neovascularization in a randomized, multicenter European phase II trial [30]. After additional treatment with GS101 eye drops, (**b**) there is marked regression of corneal neovessels compared to baseline (**a**)

Summary for the Clinician

- Current treatment options for actively growing corneal vessels include steroids, anti-VEGFs, and anti-IRS-1 eye drops.
- Anti-VEGFs such as Avastin and Lucentis given as eye drops reliably block active corneal neovascularization and also minimize vessel diameters of remaining vessels.
- Main side effects of topical anti-VEGF therapy at the ocular surface are neurotoxicity as well as delayed epithelial and stromal wound healing.
- Anti-IRS-1 eye drops given twice daily have been shown in phase II trial to safely and effectively inhibit corneal neovascularization.
- Main treatment option for mature feeder vessels is fine needle diathermy combined with topical anti-VEGFs. Main drawback is the high rate of reperfusion if disease is still active.

Treatment Options for Mature Corneal Vessels

Angioregressive therapies allow to regress preformed pathologic corneal blood vessels. Whereas the regression of novel, newly outgrown blood vessels (in the so-called "pruning-phase" [31]) can be achieved by removal of angiogenic agents such as VEGF, older and more mature and pericyte-covered vessels do not depend on angiogenic signaling any longer [31]. Induction of regression of these mature vessels is more complex, and would have to involve anti-VEGF strategies combined with agonists of the vascular endothelial TIE2 receptor (Angiopoetin 2). The regression phase for immature vessels again is very short, so that, e.g., removal of a loose suture or a hypoxia-inducing contact lens has to be performed very early after the onset of vessel outgrowths to cause regression of the new vessels. Since the mechanisms responsible for maintenance of lymphatic vessels are poorly understood, so

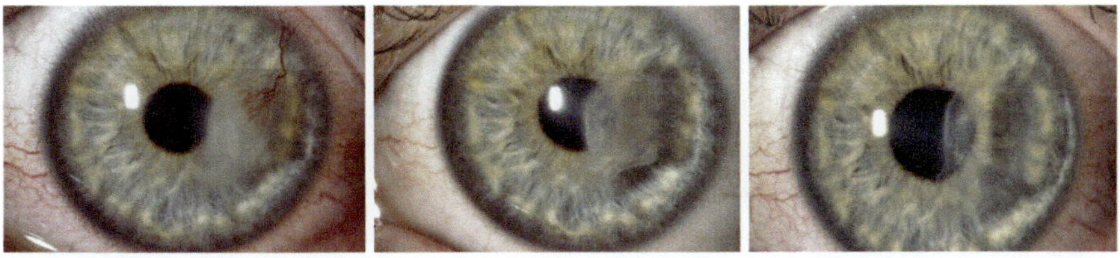

Fig. 5.7 Combined fine needle diathermy with subconjunctival Avastin and postoperative topical Avastin eye drops reliably occludes large mature feeder vessels prior to transplantation. This "preconditioning" should promote subsequent corneal graft survival [34]. *Left*: preoperatively; *middle*: 1 month after cautery and Avastin subconjunctivally and *right*: after 15 months

far no approach to pharmacologically regress lymphatic corneal vessels is known. Fortunately, lymphatic vessels in the cornea seem to regress spontaneously after the (inflammatory) stimulus subsides [22]. *Angioocclusive* approaches are useful, e.g. to prevent intraoperative bleeding during keratoplasty in vascularized high-risk eyes or to stop leakage into the cornea out of these blood vessels and to "precondition" such corneas for subsequent keratoplasty. Besides the more experimental approach of corneal photodynamic therapy, fine needle diathermy is a reliable, cost-effective, and quick treatment option. Corneal vessels are either directly cauterized or a suture needle is placed into/next to the vessel and the needle tip is then cauterized [32]. By combining that therapy with subconjunctival anti-VEGFs (e.g., Avastin) and postoperative Avastin eye drops (5 mg/ml; 5x/day for 10 days), the recurrence rate can be reduced significantly ([34]; Fig. 5.7).

Safety Profile of Anti-VEGFs at the Ocular Surface

What about the safety of topical neutralization of VEGF at the ocular surface? Although the limited evidence from published off-label clinical use of anti-VEGF therapies (primarily Bevacizumab) as well as from in vivo and in vitro safety studies suggest this specific antiangiogenic approach to be safe, several potential complications have to be kept in mind and observed thoroughly in futures studies. If one deducts potential side effects from the known physiological functions of VEGF in the cornea or in the anterior segment of the eye, several potential side effects come into play, especially given the "non-angiogenic" effects of VEGF that is its neurotrophic effect, its role in wound healing and inflammation:

(a) "Neurotrophic keratopathy": the cornea is one of the most densely innervated tissues of the human body and we know now that VEGF is a potent neurotrophic growth factor. Physiologically, there is trace amounts of VEGF found in normal avascular corneas so that VEGF in that avascular cornea also might have a neurotrophic effect. Therefore, it may well be that a long-term anti-VEGF strategy at the cornea may reduce corneal innervation, thus leading to neurotrophic keratopathy or impaired corneal nerve regeneration.

(b) "Altered immune responses": we know that VEGF is a potent chemoattractant for inflammatory cells and an essential component of the "immune amplification cascade" leading to a robust inflammatory response in the cornea. Anti-VEGF strategies may alter that ability to mount an effective immune response.
(c) "Wound healing problems": Wound healing problems are a well known side effect of angiogenesis inhibitors in vascularized tissues. But even in the avascular cornea, VEGF may play a role in wound healing. Corneal epithelium, e.g., expresses VEGFR3, which besides neutralizing VEGF-C and -D, and thus maintaining corneal angiogenic privilege, may also have an effect on epithelial proliferation. In addition, VEGFs known effect on recruitment of inflammatory cells, especially macrophages may alter corneal stromal wound healing.

Unmet Needs and Future Directions

The are numerous unmet medical needs in the management of corneal neovascularization (CN), in the scientific understanding of disease mechanisms involved in CN, and in proposing consensual approaches for the development of new drugs in this field in terms of inclusion criteria and clinical endpoints to be considered as clinically relevant. A recent consensus statement lists all current unmet needs in that field [33].

References

1. Cursiefen C, Chen L, Dana MR, Streilein JW (2003) Corneal lymphangiogenesis: evidence, mechanisms, and implications for corneal transplant immunology. Cornea 22:273–281
2. Streilein JW (2003) Ocular immune privilege: therapeutic opportunities from an experiment of nature. Nat Rev Immunol 3:879–889
3. Cursiefen C, Maruyama K, Bock F, Saban D, Sadrai Z, Lawler J, Dana R, Masli S (2011) Thrombospondin 1 inhibits inflammatory lymphangiogenesis by CD36 ligation on monocytes. J Exp Med 208:1083–1092
4. Cursiefen C, Masli S, Ng TF, Dana MR, Bornstein P, Lawler J, Streilein JW (2004) Roles of thrombospondin-1 and -2 in regulating corneal and iris angiogenesis. Invest Ophthalmol Vis Sci 45:1117–1124
5. Chen L, Hamrah P, Cursiefen C, Zhang Q, Pytowski B, Streilein JW, Dana MR (2004) Vascular endothelial growth factor receptor-3 mediates induction of corneal alloimmunity. Nat Med 10: 813–815
6. Collin HB (1966) Endothelial cell lined lymphatics in the vascularized rabbit cornea. Invest Ophthalmol 5:337–354
7. Cursiefen C, Chen L, Borges LP, Jackson D, Cao J, Radziejewski C, D'Amore PA, Dana MR, Wiegand SJ, Streilein JW (2004) VEGF-A stimulates lymphangiogenesis and hemangiogenesis in inflammatory neovascularization via macrophage recruitment. J Clin Invest 113:1040–1050
8. Cursiefen C, Schlotzer-Schrehardt U, Kuchle M, Sorokin L, Breiteneder-Geleff S, Alitalo K, Jackson D (2002) Lymphatic vessels in vascularized human corneas: immunohistochemical investigation using LYVE-1 and podoplanin. Invest Ophthalmol Vis Sci 43:2127–2135
9. Cursiefen C, Cao J, Chen L, Liu Y, Maruyama K, Jackson D, Kruse FE, Wiegand SJ, Dana MR, Streilein JW (2004) Inhibition of hemangiogenesis and lymphangiogenesis after normal-risk corneal transplantation by neutralizing VEGF promotes graft survival. Invest Ophthalmol Vis Sci 45:2666–2673

10. Dietrich T, Bock F, Yuen D, Hos D, Bachmann BO, Zahn G, Wiegand S, Chen L, Cursiefen C (2010) Cutting edge: lymphatic vessels, not blood vessels, primarily mediate immune rejections after transplantation. J Immunol 184:535–539
11. Chang JH, Gabison EE, Kato T, Azar DT (2001) Corneal neovascularization. Curr Opin Ophthalmol 12:242–249
12. Cursiefen C, Chen L, Saint-Geniez M, Hamrah P, Jin Y, Rashid S, Pytowski B, Persaud K, Wu Y, Streilein JW, Dana R (2006) Nonvascular VEGF receptor 3 expression by corneal epithelium maintains avascularity and vision. Proc Natl Acad Sci USA 103:11405–11410
13. Regenfuss B, Bock F, Parthasarathy A, Cursiefen C (2008) Corneal (lymph)angiogenesis – from bedside to bench and back: a tribute to Judah Folkman. Lymphat Res Biol 6:191–201
14. Cursiefen C, Ikeda S, Nishina PM, Smith RS, Ikeda A, Jackson D, Mo JS, Chen L, Dana MR, Pytowski B, Kruse FE, Streilein JW (2005) Spontaneous corneal hem- and lymphangiogenesis in mice with destrin-mutation depend on VEGFR3 signaling. Am J Pathol 166:1367–1377
15. Cursiefen C, Wenkel H, Martus P, Langenbucher A, Nguyen NX, Seitz B, Kuchle M, Naumann GO (2001) Impact of short-term versus long-term topical steroids on corneal neovascularization after non-high-risk keratoplasty. Graefes Arch Clin Exp Ophthalmol 239:514–521
16. Cursiefen C, Rummelt C, Kuchle M (2000) Immunohistochemical localization of vascular endothelial growth factor, transforming growth factor alpha, and transforming growth factor beta1 in human corneas with neovascularization. Cornea 19:526–533
17. Maguire MG, Stark WJ, Gottsch JD, Stulting RD, Sugar A, Fink NE, Schwartz A (1994) Risk factors for corneal graft failure and rejection in the collaborative corneal transplantation studies. Collaborative Corneal Transplantation Studies Research Group. Ophthalmology 101: 1536–1547
18. Bachmann B, Taylor RS, Cursiefen C (2010) Corneal neovascularization as a risk factor for graft failure and rejection after keratoplasty: an evidence-based meta-analysis. Ophthalmology 117:1300–1305, e1307
19. Cursiefen C, Martus P, Nguyen NX, Langenbucher A, Seitz B, Kuchle M (2002) Corneal neovascularization after nonmechanical versus mechanical corneal trephination for non-high-risk keratoplasty. Cornea 21:648–652
20. Bachmann BO, Bock F, Wiegand SJ, Maruyama K, Dana MR, Kruse FE, Luetjen-Drecoll E, Cursiefen C (2008) Promotion of graft survival by vascular endothelial growth factor a neutralization after high-risk corneal transplantation. Arch Ophthalmol 126:71–77
21. Saharinen P, Tammela T, Karkkainen MJ, Alitalo K (2004) Lymphatic vasculature: development, molecular regulation and role in tumor metastasis and inflammation. Trends Immunol 25: 387–395
22. Cursiefen C, Maruyama K, Jackson DG, Streilein JW, Kruse FE (2006) Time course of angiogenesis and lymphangiogenesis after brief corneal inflammation. Cornea 25:443–447
23. Yamagami S, Dana MR (2001) The critical role of lymph nodes in corneal alloimmunization and graft rejection. Invest Ophthalmol Vis Sci 42:1293–1298
24. Yamagami S, Dana MR, Tsuru T (2002) Draining lymph nodes play an essential role in alloimmunity generated in response to high-risk corneal transplantation. Cornea 21:405–409
25. Dietrich T, Onderka J, Bock F, Kruse FE, Vossmeyer D, Stragies R, Zahn G, Cursiefen C (2007) Inhibition of inflammatory lymphangiogenesis by integrin alpha5 blockade. Am J Pathol 171:361–372
26. Bock F, Onderka J, Dietrich T, Bachmann B, Pytowski B, Cursiefen C (2008) Blockade of VEGFR3-signalling specifically inhibits lymphangiogenesis in inflammatory corneal neovascularisation. Graefes Arch Clin Exp Ophthalmol 246:115–119
27. Hos D, Saban DR, Bock F, Regenfuss B, Onderka J, Masli S, Cursiefen C (2011) Suppression of inflammatory corneal lymphangiogenesis by application of topical corticosteroids. Arch Ophthalmol 129:445–452
28. Bock F, Onderka J, Dietrich T, Bachmann B, Kruse FE, Paschke M, Zahn G, Cursiefen C (2007) Bevacizumab as a potent inhibitor of inflammatory corneal angiogenesis and lymphangiogenesis. Invest Ophthalmol Vis Sci 48:2545–2552
29. Bock F, Konig Y, Kruse F, Baier M, Cursiefen C (2008) Bevacizumab (Avastin) eye drops inhibit corneal neovascularization. Graefes Arch Clin Exp Ophthalmol 246:281–284

30. Cursiefen C, Bock F, Horn FK, Kruse FE, Seitz B, Borderie V, Fruh B, Thiel MA, Wilhelm F, Geudelin B, Descohand I, Steuhl KP, Hahn A, Meller D (2009) GS-101 antisense oligonucleotide eye drops inhibit corneal neovascularization: interim results of a randomized phase II trial. Ophthalmology 116:1630–1637
31. Cursiefen C, Hofmann-Rummelt C, Kuchle M, Schlotzer-Schrehardt U (2003) Pericyte recruitment in human corneal angiogenesis: an ultrastructural study with clinicopathological correlation. Br J Ophthalmol 87:101–106
32. Pillai CT, Dua HS, Hossain P (2000) Fine needle diathermy occlusion of corneal vessels. Invest Ophthalmol Vis Sci 41:2148–2153
33. Cursiefen C, Colin J, Dana R, Diaz-Llopis M, Faraj L, Garcia-Delpech S, Geerling G, Price F, Remeijer L, Rouse B, Seitz B, Udaondo P, Meller D, Dua H (2012) Consensus statement on indications for anti-angiogenic therapy in the management of corneal diseases associated with neovascularisation: outcome of an expert roundtable. Br J Ophthalmol 96:3–9
34. Koenig Y, Bock F, Kruse FE, Stock K, Cursiefen C (2012) Angioregressive Pretreatment of Mature Corneal Blood Vessels Before Keratoplasty: Fine-Needle Vessel Coagulation Combined With Anti-VEGFs. Cornea Feb 22. [Epub ahead of print]
35. Steven P, Bock F, Hüttmann G, Cursiefen C (2011) Intravital two-photon microscopy of immune cell dynamics in corneal lymphatic vessels. PLoS One 6(10):e26253. Epub 2011 Oct 20

Storage of Donor Cornea for Penetrating and Lamellar Transplantation

6

Elisabeth Pels and Graeme Pollock

Core Messages

- The foundations of eye banking and corneal preservation were laid by Filatov in 1937 [1] with the recognition that donor tissue for corneal transplants could be recovered post-mortem.
- Over the past few decades the responsibility for the provision of a viable, disease-free donor cornea has been entrusted to the eye bank, and the ophthalmic surgeon now has to rely on these services as an important aspect of their surgery and treatment.
- With the appreciation that corneal transplantation could potentially transmit a number of diseases from donor to recipient, eye banks became increasingly responsible for donor screening for such diseases and standards to assist in these practices were developed.
- Today, eye banking services are provided in an environment of stringent quality assurance standards, often with increasing government regulation or oversight. Quality management systems and risk assessment have become important aspects of eye banking where the emphasis is now not only on quantity of tissue provided but also where quality of tissue and quality of service have become priorities.

E. Pels, Ph.D. (✉)
Cornea Bank Amsterdam, Euro Tissue Bank,
Markt 58, 1941 BM Beverwijk, The Netherlands
e-mail: epels@eurotissuebank.nl; e.pels@hetnet.nl

G. Pollock, Ph.D.
Lions Eye Donation Service Melbourne, Royal Victorian Eye and Ear Hospital,
32 Gisborne Street, 3002 Melbourne, VIC, Australia
e-mail: graemeap@unimelb.edu.au

T. Reinhard, F. Larkin (eds.), *Corneal Disease*,
DOI 10.1007/978-3-642-28747-3_6, © Springer-Verlag Berlin Heidelberg 2013

- Different recovery procedures, storage techniques, and in more recent years, tissue processing techniques, have been introduced and each have their own benefits and risks in regard to their technical, microbiological and tissue evaluation aspects.
- Eye bank preparation of donor tissue for lamellar endothelial keratoplasty procedures is evolving rapidly but presents unique challenges to the eye bank, especially in regard to handling and iatrogenic damage during processing.

Introduction

The foundations of eye banking and corneal preservation were laid by Filatov in 1937 with the recognition that donor tissue for corneal transplants could be recovered post-mortem [1]. For many years, the ophthalmic surgeon was in direct control of the process, often being directly responsible for both procurement of donor tissue and the transplant surgery itself. However, over the past few decades, the responsibility for the provision of a viable, disease-free donor cornea has been entrusted to the eye bank, and the ophthalmic surgeons now have to rely on these services as an important aspect of their surgery and treatment.

The first eye bank was perhaps the Eye Bank for Sight Restoration in New York, founded in 1944. At this time, eye banks functioned as collection centres and simple storage facilities, holding whole globes in moist pot storage prior to corneal transplantation, which was usually undertaken within 24 h of donor eye retrieval. Eye banking practices expanded during the 1970s with the development of corneoscleral storage solutions [2] which allowed, for several days, storage and the refinement of corneal evaluation procedures to determine the suitability and likely efficacy of a cornea for a particular transplant procedure. Such activity helped support the rapid growth of corneal transplantation over the same period which was being driven by advances in instrumentation, surgical microscopy and suture development. Accompanying such growth was the appreciation that corneal transplantation could potentially transmit a number of diseases from donor to recipient, and eye banks became increasingly responsible for donor screening for such diseases [3]. Many of the standards to assist in these practices were initially developed by the Eye Bank Association of America (EBAA, www.restoresight.org) who produced their first set of Medical Standards in 1980. These standards are maintained and updated by rigorous and regular review processes. Other Eye Banks and Eye Banking associations, such as the European Eye Bank Association (EEBA, www.europeaneyebanks.com) and the Eye Bank Association of Australian and New Zealand (EBAANZ, www.ebaanz.org) have also developed their own set of Standards using those of the EBAA as their basis and cover areas such as donor selection and testing, personnel and training, facilities and equipment, documentation, procurement and corneal preservation.

Today, eye banking services are provided in an environment of stringent quality assurance standards, often with increasing government regulation or oversight. All of these systems have as their basis the identification and minimisation of risk so as to ensure and improve the quality and safety of transplanted tissue. Quality management systems and risk assessment have become important aspects of eye banking where the emphasis is now not only on quantity of tissue provided but also where quality of tissue and quality of service have become priorities.

Different recovery procedures, storage techniques, and in more recent years tissue processing techniques, have been introduced and each have their own benefits and risks. These will be compared in this chapter. However, the adoption or choice of a particular procedure needs to be considered within the context of a practitioner's local conditions to ensure an efficient, safe and quality service. Ultimately, the objective of eye banking remains – the delivery of ocular tissue, donated for transplantation, in order to allow the ophthalmic surgeon to restore sight in a safe and high-quality procedure.

Retrieval of Donor Tissue

Either the corneoscleral button is removed in situ and directly transferred to a storage or collection solution, or the eye is enucleated and the corneoscleral button excised later in the eye bank laboratory. Legal requirements will vary between jurisdictions, with some legislature requiring that only medical practitioners be authorised to perform the donor procedure, and still some others specifying that only in situ excision rather than enucleation be allowed. The suggested procedures for enucleation and in situ excision are described in the Medical and Technical Standards of many eye banks and eye banking organisations. Ultimately, the preferred method is dependent on local/national conditions and considerations and legalities but the persons performing the donor surgery must use their professional judgment and satisfy themselves that all reasonable steps and normal surgical precautions have been taken to minimise contamination or damage to the tissue.

Technical Aspects

The benefits and risks of both procedures are summarised in Table 6.1. In situ excision is more technically demanding and also requires the time to perform a careful in situ examination by penlight or handheld slit lamp. The introduction of the artificial anterior chamber also means that lamellar surgical techniques can be performed on the corneoscleral button obviating need for a whole eye. The enucleation procedure is more invasive with the risk of haemorrhages from the optic vessels and the orbit affecting the appearance of the donor, although this is not a common problem [4].

Upon the death of the donor, the corneal endothelium is subject to warm ischemia and is in contact with stagnant aqueous humour. This results in progressive cytolysis and cell death and this may also progress during subsequent storage.

Table 6.1 Tissue retrieval considerations

Factors to consider		In situ excision	Enucleation
Legal provisions		Tissue removal	Organ removal
Technical procedure	Staff	Medical/technical trained	Trained
	Time	Longer	Shorter
	Risk	Less invasive	Risk of haemorrhage
Eye bank facility		Not necessary	Laboratory
Contamination rate		Similar to higher in organ culture	
Tissue evaluation		Pen light, slit lamp	Slit lamp
Inspection anterior chamber		Pen light	Slit lamp
Tissue viability		Similar or better due to shorter delay expiration–excision	

Limiting the time between the cessation of donor circulation and storage of the cornea results in a more viable endothelium, but an absolute acceptable time interval has not yet been defined. Recommended death to enucleation times for corneas intended for organ culture storage tend to be more liberal than those for hypothermic storage. The normothermic temperatures of organ culture storage provide for an in-built viability assay on the "health" of the cornea, and evaluation at the end of the storage period allows for a discard of those corneas they may have suffered from ischaemic damage following the donor's death. A period of 24 h (or beyond) death to enucleation is often a recommended benchmark. Conversely, hypothermic storage doesn't provide for this type of assessment and thus more conservative maximum death to enucleation times of 12–18 h are often used as a benchmark.

Microbiological Aspects

The normal ocular flora that is present during life multiplies with the lack of lid movement and lyzosomal enzymes in the tear film. Before removal of the tissue, bacterial contamination from both exogenous sources and from the ocular flora post-mortem [5] has to be removed. For in situ excision, one must be especially aware of the bacteriologic considerations, as no further decontamination of the tissue is possible. In general, the procedure consists of vigorous rinsing with balanced salt solution, moistening of the eye and eye lashes with a broad-spectrum antibiotic/antifungal solution and disinfection of the lids and the surrounding eye tissue and skin with povidone–iodine solution. In the case of enucleation, many eye banks will forego extensive donor preparation, opting instead to decontaminate the globe within the laboratory. This is usually done by vigorous rinsing with a balanced salt solution, immersion of the eye in a 0.5–1% povidone–iodine solution, followed by a subsequent rinse with balanced salt (See technical guidelines EBAA, EBAANZ and EEBA). Comparative studies support the validity of both procedures [5].

The overall rate of post-operative endophthalmitis following penetrating keratoplasty has been found to be around 0.4% in a literature review of 90,549 cases [6].

These rates have been decreasing over the last decade and this has been ascribed to improved eye banking procedures. However, surgeons need to be made aware of the microbiological condition of the received donor tissue. This may include information regarding the risk of tissue contamination, the decontamination steps and measures taken during processing, the storage procedure, the antibiotics that may have been used and the results of any microbiological tests that may have been performed (see section on corneal storage).

Tissue Evaluation Aspects

Enucleation allows for a more extensive anterior segment evaluation by a slit lamp, while examination in situ examination is often limited by the use of a penlight. This examination is important to determine if there has been previous anterior segment surgery or if there is any pathology of the eye that may not have been identified through the donor screening process. However, the examination of the excised cornea in the eye bank laboratory is possible by the slit lamp. The endothelium is the primary layer responsible for the maintenance of corneal hydration and transparency. Tests to assess the functional capacity of the endothelium cannot be applied during eye banking as they affect corneal viability. Therefore, one has to rely on the morphology of the endothelium to reflect its functional reserve and routine inspection of the endothelium is nowadays part of the donor evaluation. Assessment of the cornea by biomicroscopy of the endothelium also provides a quantifiable means of determining suitability for use and helps to increase the donor supply by objectively assessing corneas that may otherwise be arbitrarily excluded for transplantation beforehand on the basis of, for example, age or post-mortem time. While studies linking graft outcome with morphometric parameters of the endothelium are lacking, models to calculate cell loss over extended periods after penetrating keratoplasty have been presented [7, 8]. They provide a rationale for accepting a minimum donor cell density. Many eye banks consider about 2,000 cells/mm^2 to be a minimum in cases of where transplantation of the endothelium is involved. In addition, an endothelial layer with considerable polymegathism or pleomorphism and/or the presence of guttae is considered indicative of a cornea that may be functionally deficient or compromised [9]. Ultimately, however, the final decision regarding use rests with the surgeon for each individual patient transplant procedure undertaken while taking the Eye Bank's evaluation report into account.

Corneal Storage

For the whole eye, the most common storage method is moistened pot or moist chamber storage at 2–6°C, introduced in 1937 [1]. Today this technique is usually a temporary holding or transport method that precedes corneoscleral button excision.

Today the prevailing storage methods are those of placing the corneoscleral button in a modified tissue culture medium. The cornea is then stored hypothermically at 2–6°C, a method introduced in 1974 by Mc Carey and Kaufman, or

Table 6.2 Storage procedures for the corneoscleral button

Factors to consider	Hypothermic	Organ culture
Technique	Simple and fast	More complex
	Minimal handling	
Storage time	Up to 10 days	Up to 4–7 weeks
Tissue available for direct use	Yes	No
Maintenance hydration	Yes	No
		Reversal swelling necessary
Epithelial and endothelial wound healing	No	Yes
	More strict concerning donor supply	More tolerant for conditions affecting endothelial viability
Evaluation tissue technique	Non-invasive	Invasive
	Specular microscope (invasive light microscopy)	Light microscopy
Evaluation endothelium	Small central area	Entire surface
Risk primary graft failure	Overall reported mean 2%	0–0.3%
	Currently estimated 1%	
	Greater when storage time > 7 days	
Graft survival		At least comparable
Microbiological tests	Not required	Mandatory
		Quarantine period
		More tolerant for septicaemic risk donor
Risk of post-operative endophthalmitis	0.1–2%	0–0.1%
Storage solutions	Commercial available	Commercial available/ in-house manufacture

normothermically at 30–37°C, the "organ culture" method introduced in 1976 by Doughman. These techniques require good asepsis and careful application, and increasingly, eye banks are implementing quality assurance programs for good tissue banking practice to ensure the quality and validity of processes. The different storage procedures for the corneoscleral button are summarised in Table 6.2. Although some success has been reported with corneas frozen in liquid nitrogen, it is not a generally accepted storage method for corneas.

Moist Chamber Storage of the Donor Eye

Technical Aspects

The enucleated eye is placed in a sealed chamber together with gauze, moistened with saline or an antibiotic solution and stored at 2–6°C. Immersion in the saline solution must be prevented to avoid the cornea taking up extraneous fluid that would result in epithelial and stromal oedema.

Storage Period

As part of the globe, the corneal endothelium is in contact with the stagnant aqueous humour. Accordingly, necrotising tissue, metabolic waste products and hydrolytic enzymes accumulate with time. Since these are toxic for the endothelium, the storage time is limited to 48–72 h.

The storage time of the whole eye generally does not exceed 24 h prior to corneoscleral button excision and storage.

Microbiological Safety

The effectiveness of antibiotic solutions in reducing microbial flora and contamination is debatable since their effectiveness at low temperatures cannot be verified. However, antibiotics may accumulate in the tissue and may be an effective prophylaxis following transplant surgery.

Tissue Evaluation

The slit lamp is the usual method of evaluating the cornea. This can be supplemented with examination of the endothelium by specular microscopy provided the cornea is not too swollen and therefore it needs to be performed as soon as possible after retrieval surgery.

Hypothermic Storage of the Corneoscleral Button

Technical Aspects

The corneoscleral buttons are placed in a modified tissue culture solution and stored at 2–6°C. Handling of the cornea is minimised as the evaluation of the endothelium by slit lamp and specular microscopy is usually performed with the cornea remaining in its container. The formula for some older storage solutions, such as M-K [2] are in the published literature while the more modern storage solutions are commercially available. Storage parameters such as temperature and maximum time of storage vary between solutions and need to be followed as prescribed. The corneoscleral buttons are directly available for surgery provided that the donor's medical history and tissue serology permits release.

The fundamental composition of hypothermic storage solutions is tissue culture medium supplemented with antibiotics and an osmotic agent such as dextran to compensate for the inactivity of the cornea's normal water removal mechanism at 4°C, thus preventing cell swelling and maintaining corneal deturgescence. More modern variants have increased storage times through the addition of energy sources, antioxidants, membrane stabilising factors and growth factors. Most importantly, the addition of chondroitin sulphate has provided better endothelial cell viability during storage while also acting as an additional osmotic agent, extending acceptable storage times [2]. However, degenerative changes in the endothelium as a result of post-mortem time and other variables such as cause and circumstances of death will progress during hypothermic storage and thus limit storage times. In addition, epithelial healing at hypothermic temperatures is not possible and indeed the epithelium can be compromised when the hypothermic storage is prolonged [10]. To reduce these risks, the recommended storage periods are kept far below the original reported maxima and the benchmark time interval from death to storage of the corneoscleral button is often kept well within 12 h.

Storage Period

The original M-K medium was reported to provide a safe storage period up to 10 days, although the generally accepted period in practice is limited to 3–4 days. Some of the later introduced storage solutions such as K-sol, Dexsol, Likorol, Optisol (GS) report longer periods and storage for 7–10 days is generally accepted.

Microbiological Safety

The reported overall incidence of postoperative keratitis and ophthalmitis caused by microbes transferred with the cornea varies from 0.1% to 2% [11]. This is despite reported figures of positive donor rims of up to 19% [12], indicating that the antibiotics in storage solutions cannot be very effective at these low temperatures of storage. Instead it can be assumed that, upon return to physiological temperature, the residual antibiotic effect in the donor cornea coupled with the recipient's ocular immune defense normally proves to be sufficient to control any organisms.

Tissue Evaluation

Non-invasive specular microscopy of the endothelium (coupled with slit lamp examination) is the favoured method for evaluating hypothermically stored corneas. Indeed, since 2001, determination of the endothelial cell density is required by the Medical Standards of the EEBA. Most specular microscopes are today equipped with software programmes to determine parameters such as cell count, variation in cell size, cell shape although careful calibration needs to be performed to obtain reliable morphometric results [13].

A limitation with specular microscopy is that the area of the central corneal endothelium is much larger than can be sampled by the specular microscope even with multiple field examinations. Therefore, the information gained from specular microscopy must be interpreted within the context of the slit lamp evaluation. In addition, the best observation of the corneal endothelium is at room temperature after the placement of the cornea in storage media, yet allowing sufficient time for adequate deturgescence of the cornea necessary to view the endothelial cells [9]. Therefore, degenerative changes and possible endothelial cell loss during storage, which may result in inferior quality and/or primary graft failure, cannot always be readily evaluated, but it must be taken into account [14, 15].

The incidence of primary graft failure has been reported to be between 0% and 10% and is currently believed to be about 1% [15]. Evaluation of the endothelium may reduce the risk of primary graft failure and increase long-term graft survival, but studies supporting this premise are lacking. However, examination of the endothelium certainly plays a role in setting higher and more uniform standards and helps to increase the donor supply by assessing corneas that may otherwise be arbitrarily excluded for transplantation on basis of donor age or previous ocular surgery.

Organ Culture (Normothermic Storage) of the Corneoscleral Button

Technical Aspects

The corneosclereal buttons are stored in an incubator at 30–37°C. The procedure was developed by Doughman (1976), modified by Sperling(1979) and further developed and refined in Europe [16]. The technique provides storage of the corneoscleral buttons up to 4–6 weeks or even longer.

The technique is more complex compared to hypothermic storage. It requires microbiological surveillance during storage and mandatory evaluation of the endothelium at the end of the storage period. In addition, the storage solution, consisting of tissue culture medium, foetal bovine serum as source for energy, proteins, growth factors and antibiotics, does not contain macromolecules to maintain corneal hydration in vitro [16]. This swelling of the cornea is reversed before surgery by transfer of the tissue to a dextran-supplemented storage medium (referred to as the Transport or Thinning medium) [16]. This later medium is also used to transport the cornea (conveniently) at room temperature. Due to the number of steps involved in organ culture storage, relative to hypothermic storage, the cornea is not directly available for surgery.

Storage Period

The storage time in the organ culture medium may be up to 4–7 weeks after excision. Renewal of the medium during storage (at 10–14 days) may promote an extended storage time [16].

Depending on the eye bank, reported maximum times for the cornea placed in transport medium vary from 1 to 7 days and the dextran concentration varies from 4% to 8%. This largely determines the extent of the reversal of corneal swelling (usually to a level dependent on the preference of the recipient surgeons). Time spent in transport medium is limited by the toxic effects of dextran over time, which is ingested in cellular vacuoles [16].

Microbiological Safety

The antibiotics present in the storage solution are effective during organ culture. In the absence of antibiotics and despite extensive corneal decontamination before organ culture, the corneas themselves have been responsible for greater than 30% microbial contamination of cultures [16]. Even in the presence of antibiotics, the organ culture mediuma remains a highly nutrient medium for the continued growth of any contaminating organisms. Thus, microbiological testing and surveillance of the storage solution is mandatory and a quarantine period for the corneas is required until the results of microbiological testing of the culture solution are available. Any contaminated organ cultures are discarded. When these procedures are followed, the reported incidence of endophthalmitis from corneas transplanted after organ culture is 0–0.1% (EEBA Directory).

The rate of contaminated cultures varies between eye banks. It appears to be dependent on several variables: the antibiotic cocktail in the medium (narrow- to wide-spectrum antibiotics), in situ excision or enucleation, and the post-mortem delay between death of the donor and collection and storage (EEBA Directory). Most importantly, organ culture may become the method of choice when corneas are suspected to be contaminated, for example, from a donor with bacteraemia [17]. The storage itself acts as an in-built microbiological surveillance system, since any culture containing microorganisms not controlled by decontamination and antibiotics will become contaminated, and the cornea not used for transplant.

Tissue Evaluation

Although mandatory only after storage, inspection of the endothelium is often performed both before and after storage (EEBA Directory). Differences in endothelial cell loss in individual corneas may occur as a result of wound healing processes and impaired endothelial viability due to post mortem time, cause and circumstances of death, etc. In this way, organ culture might be considered as a stress test or an in-built viability test for the cornea. Corneas showing significant cell loss will be discarded before surgery [16]. Interestingly, 100% cell loss has been found associated with a herpes infection [18].

The specular microscope is not suitable for the inspection of organ-cultured corneas as it requires an un-swollen cornea. Therefore, the endothelium of organ-cultured corneas is generally assessed by light microscopy together with vital dye staining. These methods were developed along with the introduction of the organ culture procedure in Europe [19]. It allows the inspection of the entire endothelial surface irrespective of the corneal thickness and transparency. In addition, the use of the vital dye trypan blue allows the detection of non-viable cells and denuded Descemet's membrane. The method is invasive and requires the use of hypotonic solutions to temporarily swell the intracellular spaces so that the endothelial cells can be visualised. This must be done using aseptic conditions. It is variously performed (depending on the eye bank) as a bright field microscope or a phase contrast image using inverted or non-inverted microscopes. The induction and the swelling pattern are dependent on storage time and medium and therefore, interpretation of the images requires experience and standardised working conditions.

For parameters such as cell counts, some type of image analysis is required. The light microscope set up needs to be well-calibrated for these purposes [20]. Modern image software aims for automated cell analysis that is independent of the observer and experience. However, so far, reliable results can only be obtained after much time-consuming interactive manipulation which requires experienced observers. Confocal microscopy is a promising development for future analysis of eye bank corneas but it awaits the development of a non-contact version for eye banking for it to gain widespread acceptance.

Other Aspects

Organ-cultured corneas are evaluated at the end of the storage period and therefore eye banks using this technique have less limitations in regard to post-mortem to enucleation and excision times (EEBA Directory). This also serves to increase the potential donor pool.

The reported incidence of primary graft failure of corneas stored by organ culture is low at 0–0.3% [EEBA Directory].

Organ culture is a method best suited to an established eye bank with skilled technical staff, and where donor rates are variable, or where distribution is required over wide geographical area. In addition, Europe has preferred the technique because the increased storage time allows the ability to provide ABO- or HLA-matched corneas for patients with high risk of rejection, and for optimising allocation of particular corneas to specific patients.

Pre-cutting of Corneal Tissue for Endothelial Keratoplasty (EK)

Over the past decade, endothelial transplant procedures have evolved to a point where they have become a preferred method of surgical treatment for endothelial dysfunction. There have been a number of variations in the procedure, and thus variants in donor tissue preparation, over this time. Currently, the primary preparations are Descemet's Stripping EK (DSEK) which involves manual surgical dissection and preparation of the donor lenticule, and its subtype Descemet's Stripping Automated EK (DSAEK) which introduces microkeratome preparation of the donor lenticule [21, 22]. More recently, Descemet's Membrane EK (DMEK), where the endothelium with Descemet's membrane in the absence of any stroma is transplanted, has been introduced and it presents its own unique set of difficulties in donor tissue preparation [23].

The preparation of donor lenticules by the eye banks (pre-cut tissue) introduced a number of major advantages over surgeon preparation of tissue [22]). Importantly, the eye bank is able to evaluate the tissue quality of the donor posterior lenticule by (specular) microscopy, slit lamp biomicroscopy and (more recently) by optical coherence tomography [24] immediately post-resection. This allows for the exclusion of any donor lenticules that may have been compromised by the cutting or dissection procedure. It also reduces the time spent by the surgeon in preparing the tissue and saves operating room time. Indeed, eye bank staff can also become extremely proficient at the procedure due to high volumes of procedures which results in more consistent resection outcomes. Although the use of eye bank-prepared donor tissue simplifies EK, the ophthalmic surgeon must once again rely on the eye bank personnel to reliably perform a critical portion of the procedure. In addition, there is concern that adverse tissue changes may occur between the extended time when the tissue is pre-cut and the time the tissue is transplanted, including swelling of the lenticule due to exposure of stromal tissue to storage media and possible loss of endothelial cells [25]. However, these concerns about eye bank pre-cut tissue appear to be unfounded with reported transplant outcomes similar to that of surgeon-prepared tissue [22].

Both manual dissection and microkeratome cutting are used by eye banks in providing pre-cut tissue, and femtosecond laser cutting of EK lenticules is currently under development. However, all of these procedures present many significant financial, logistic and technical challenges for eye banks to undertake.

Microkeratome Cutting

The microkeratome (for DSAEK preparation) is the most common procedure employed by eye banks providing pre-cut tissue. This activity is growing rapidly – in the United States for the year 2009, 20% of EKs were performed with eye bank pre-cut tissue, whereas in 2008 this figure was less than 1% [22]. European data suggest their 2009 pre-cut use was approximately 6%. In New Zealand and parts of Australia, all DSAEK tissue is provided pre-cut by the eye bank. The slower uptake in Europe may be due to the fact that in many European countries pre-cutting is considered as engineering of the tissue by national regulatory authorities, and an upgrade to a Good Manufacturing Practice class B environment is required in order to perform the cutting.

The thickness of the lenticule produced by microkeratome cutting is dependent on the interactions between the speed of movement of the cutting head across the cornea, the head size and the degree of pressure applied within the artificial anterior chamber. Experience is required in balancing these variables to produce the required thickness. Automated microkeratomes with set drive speeds and controlled calibrated pressures reduce this flexibility in approach but in less experienced hands it may provide more consistency and predictability of the process. Microkeratome cutting produces a smoother stromal interface than manual resection, and this has been casually associated with increased dislocation rates of DSAEK compared to DSEK.

While there is now some accumulated experience and knowledge regarding DSAEK pre-cut tissue with hypothermically stored corneas, there is limited experience in using organ-cultured stored corneas. The dynamics of the swelling of the cornea during the storage phase and the reversal of the swelling in the transfer/transport phase of the technique complicate the timing and approach to a DSAEK cut. In addition, at the physiological temperatures of organ culture, the epithelium continues to grow, and down-growth of the epithelium to the cutting plane might be a risk. The effects of cutting prior to storage or prior to transfer into the transport/tinning medium are largely unknown. Limited experience of cutting after transfer and thinning (and subsequent transport) in 6% dextran medium is available (Venice Eye Bank, personal communication 2010). In Australia and New Zealand, organ cultured DSAEK corneas are cut 24 h after placement in a 5% dextran solution and short-term outcomes appear to be satisfactory, although obtaining optimal thickness of the posterior lenticule, at the time of cutting and after a period of transport, has been difficult (personal communication). The use of higher dextran concentrations to further dehydrate and thin the cornea allowing a deeper cut and a thinner lenticule, and the full effects of swelling, reversal of the swelling and transport after cutting requires further investigation.

Femtosecond Laser Cutting

Femtosecond laser preparation of donor tissue is an appealing concept since it provides bladeless computer-controlled precision cutting of the cornea with minimal adjacent stromal and endothelial cell morphological changes. The cutting plane, being "within" the cornea itself, ensures that the surfaces are not directly exposed to storage media. In theory, this reduces the risk of stromal swelling and any accompanying changes in Descemet's Membrane and endothelial cells. Bladeless cutting also eliminates the risk of epithelial cells being introduced into the cut surface and thus reduces the risk of epithelial in-growth. Corneal storage and tissue evaluation may be performed in the same way as for non-cut tissue. However, the possibility that corneal wound healing during subsequent organ culture storage could "repair" the cut needs further study.

Cheng et al. [26] showed the feasibility of the procedure for organ culture, and laboratory-based studies with hypothermically [27] and normothermically [28] stored corneas have been performed. In these studies, dissection was not always complete and required surgical intervention or a double-pass ablation to complete and allow for peeling apart of the tissue along the cutting plane. The thickness and smoothness of the surface of the lamellae was also inconsistent and was thought to be related to variations in the hydration of the deep stromal layers of the cornea. These technical difficulties are still to be overcome and may be possible, with the introduction of lasers operating at a higher Hertz and the refinement and customisation of nomograms in respect to corneal applanation and repetition rate of firing.

Stripping of Descemet's Membrane with Endothelium

Descemet's Membrane EK (DMEK) is the latest EK procedure whereby only Descemet's membrane and attached endothelium is transplanted with no attached stromal tissue. The ultrathin transplant promises accelerated and optimal visual recovery and good results have been reported by Melles and co-workers [23], and others [21]. However, the technical difficulties involved in both donor tissue preparation and delivering the donor endothelium to the participating clinic presents significant challenges with reports of an 8% increase in donor tissue wastage [23]. A specific storage and delivery device for the very thin lamellae, which by nature roll up with the endothelial layer at the outside, has been developed to provide the necessary delicate handling of the tissue [29]. Interestingly, with increasing age of the donor, the thickness of Descemet's membrane increases and the elasticity of the corneal tissue decreases. Therefore, for the preparation and handling of this kind of posterior lamellae, a higher age of the donor is preferred.

More recently, a hybrid technique of donor preparation has been described which involves removal of the Descemet's membrane endothelial lamella pneumatically from a thick posterior corneoscleral lamella previously prepared with the microkeratome termed Descemet's membrane automated EK (DMAEK). The periphery of the prepared endothelial graft remains attached to the stroma and the entire dissected corneoscleral disc is stored [30]. Complete detachment was achieved in 95% of cases, the average diameter of the bubble was 8 mm and the average loss in endothelial cell density after 7 days of storage was 4%. A small case series of ten patients has demonstrated that this preparation facilitates surgery, reduces complications and maintains good DMEK outcomes.

Donor Considerations for EK

As for any corneal transplant procedure, EK success is dependent upon the functional capacity and viability of the endothelial cells on the posterior lamella. Primary graft failure is much more common in EK than in PK and this has in some quarters been attributed to insufficient quality of the donor tissue provided for the procedure. In turn, this has led to surgeons requesting donor tissue that meets criteria in excess to that provided for PK surgery, i.e., younger donors, less storage time and higher endothelial cell densities than for PK corneas. However, over a number of publications, Terry's group has shown that there is no correlation between storage time and endothelial cell survival following DSAEK surgery, and higher donor endothelial cells counts make no difference to outcome [22]. They have identified that most primary graft failures for EK are almost certainly iatrogenic and are because of surgical trauma to the endothelium during tissue preparation, insertion and subsequent positioning.

In summary, the success of pre-cut tissue is dependent on a number of codependent factors that need to be balanced for each particular transplant:

(i) The thickness of the lamellae.
The thinner the lamellae the earlier is the visual recovery and higher percentage of patients reaching optimal visual acuity. However, these benefits come with the risk of increased manipulation of donor tissue during preparation and surgery, iatrogenic damage to the endothelium, and thus increased primary graft failures, increased reoperation rates and increased wastage of valuable donor tissue during preparation.

(ii) A regularly produced smooth cutting surface.
A smoother interface surface (e.g. DSAEK vs. DSEK) can provide better optics for vision. However, smoother surfaces also result in difficulties in getting the lamellae to adhere and lead to greater dislocation rates.

Summary for the Clinician

- The choice of a particular procedure for the retrieval of donor tissue, in situ corneoscleral excision or and enucleation, has to be considered within the context of an eye bank's local conditions to ensure an efficient, safe and quality service.
- Comparison of the different corneal storage techniques of hypothermic and normothermic organ culture, in regards to their technical, microbiological and tissue evaluation aspects shows that each technique will ensure an efficient, safe and quality service and preference is dependent on the local eye bank's conditions.
- Most experience with pre-cut tissue for lamellar grafting has been with hypothermically stored microkeratome cut corneas and with manually prepared organ-cultured corneas. This experience has helped define the necessary corneal parameters required for a good outcome. The newer techniques of femtosecond laser predissection and Descemet's membrane -endothelium complex endothelium preparations also offer great promise. Pre-cut preparation presents challenges to the eye bank, especially in regard to handling and iatrogenic damage introduced during processing.

References

1. Filatov VP (1937) Transplantation of cornea from preserved cadaver eyes. Lancet 1:1395
2. Kaufman HE (1999) Tissue storage systems: short and intermediate term. In: Brightbill FS (ed) Corneal surgery: theory, technique and practice, 3rd edn. Mosby, St. Louis, pp 892–897
3. Pollock GA, Moffatt SL (2010) Eye banking: a practical guide. In: Valparee RB (ed) Corneal transplantation, 2nd edn. Jaypee Brothers, New Delhi, pp 20–37
4. Soper MC, Lisitza MA (1999) Tissue removal. In: Brightbill FS (ed) Corneal surgery: theory, technique and practice, 3rd edn. Mosby, St. Louis, pp 882–887
5. Kim J, Kim MJ, Stoeger C et al (2010) Comparison of in situ excision and whole-globe recovery of corneal tissue in a large, single eye bank series. Am J Ophthalmol 150: 427–433
6. Taban M, Behrens A, Newcomb RL et al (2005) Incidence of acute endophthalmitis following penetrating keratoplasty; a systemic review. Arch Ophthalmol 123:605–609
7. Armitage WJ, Dick AD, Bourne WM (2003) Predicting endothelial cell loss and long term graft survival. Invest Ophthalmol Vis Sci 44:3326–3331
8. Böhringer D, Böhringer S, Poxleitner K et al (2010) Long term graft survival in penetrating keratoplasty: the biexponential model of chronic endothelial cell loss revisited. Cornea 29:1113–1117
9. Laing RA (1999) Specular microscopy. In: Brightbill FS (ed) Corneal surgery: theory, technique and practice, 3rd edn. Mosby, St. Louis, pp 101–112
10. Kim T, Palay DA, Lynn M (1996) Donor factors associated with epithelial defects after penetrating keratoplasty. Cornea 15:451–456
11. Everts RJ, Fowler WC, Chang DH et al (2001) Corneoscleral rim cultures: lack of utility and implications for clinical decision-making and infection prevention in the care of patients undergoing corneal transplantations. Cornea 20:586–589
12. Wiffen SJ, Weston BC, Maguire LJ, Bourne BM (1997) The value of routine donor corneal rim cultures in penetrating keratoplasty. Arch Ophthalmol 115:719–724
13. Van Schaick W, Van Dooren BT, Mulder PGH (2005) Validity of endothelial cell analysis methods and recommendation for calibration in Topcon SP-2000P specular microscopy. Cornea 24:538–544
14. Komuro K, Hodge DO, Gores GJ et al (1999) Cell death during corneal storage at 4°C. Invest Ophthalmol Vis Sci 40:2827–2832
15. Wilhelmus KR, Stulting D, Sugar J et al (1995) Primary corneal graft failure. A national reporting system. Arch Ophthalmol 113:1497–502
16. Pels E, Schuchard Y (1993) Organ culture and endothelial evaluation as a preservation method for human corneas. In: Brightbill FS (ed) Corneal surgery: theory, technique and practice, 2nd edn. Mosby, St. Louis, pp 622–633
17. Spelsberg H, Reinhard T, Sengler U et al (2002) Organ-cultured corneal grafts from septic donors; a retrospective study. Eye 16:622–627
18. Cleator GM, Klapper PE, Dennett C et al (1994) Corneal donor infection by herpes simplex virus: herpes simplex virus DNA in donor corneas. Cornea 13:294–304
19. Sperling S (1986) Evaluation of the endothelium of human donor corneas by induced dilation of the intercellular spaces and trypan blue. Graefes Arch Clin Exp Ophthalmol 224: 428–434
20. Thuret C, Manisolle S, Le Petit JC et al (2003) Is manual counting of corneal endothelial cell density in eye banks still acceptable? The French experience. Br J Ophthalmol 87:1481–1486
21. Price MO, Giebel AW, Fairchild KM et al (2009) Descemet membrane endothelial keratoplasty: prospective multicenter study of visual and refractive outcomes and endothelial survival. Ophthalmology 116:2361–2368
22. Terry MA (2009) Endothelial keratoplasty: a comparison of complication rats and endothelial survival between precut tissue and surgeon-cut tissue by a single DSAEK surgeon. Trans Am Ophthalmol Soc 107:184–191
23. Ham L, van Luijk C, Dapena I et al (2009) Endothelial cell density after descemet membrane endothelial keratoplasty: 1- to 2-year follow-up. Am J Ophthalmol 148:521–527

24. Brown JS, Wang D, Xiaoli L et al (2008) In situ ultrahigh-resolution optical coherence tomography characterization of eye bank corneal tissue processed for lamellar keratoplasty. Cornea 27:802–810
25. Ide T, Yoo SH, Kymionis GD et al (2008) Descemet-stripping automated endothelial keratoplasty. Effect of anterior lamellar corneal tissue-on/-off storage condition on descemet-stripping automated endothelial keratoplasty donor tissue. Cornea 27:754–757
26. Cheng YYY, Pels E, Nuijts RMMA (2007) Femtosecond-laser-assisted Descemet's stripping endothelial keratoplasty. J Cat Refrac Surg 33:152–155
27. Mehta JS, Shilbayeh R, Por YM et al (2008) Femtosecond laser creation of donor cornea buttons for Descemet-stripping endothelial keratoplasty. J Cataract Refract Surg 34:1970–1975
28. Cheng YY, Kang SJ, Grossniklaus HE (2009) Histologic evaluation of human posterior lamellar discs for femtosecond laser Descemet's stripping endothelial keratoplasty. Cornea 28: 73–79
29. Lie JT, Birbal R, Ham L et al (2008) Donor tissue preparation for Descemet membrane endothelial keratoplasty. J Cataract Refract Surg 34:1578–1583
30. Busin M, Scorcia V, Patel AK et al (2010) Pneumatic dissection and storage of donor endothelial tissue for Descemet's membrane endothelial keratoplasty: a novel technique. Ophthalmology 117:1517–1520

Infant Keratoplasty

7

Peter Kim and David S. Rootman

Core Messages

- Infant keratoplasty aims to clear the visual axis and allow for functional visual development.
- The decision to operate on an infant must be individualized and should consider the risks and benefits of surgery.
- Visual prognosis is related to severity of ocular pathology with acquired conditions generally having better outcomes than congenital indications.
- A comprehensive clinical history and examination as well as appropriate ancillary testing establishes the preoperative diagnosis, assists with surgical planning, and indicates the visual potential of the eye.
- Penetrating keratoplasty in infants is technically more difficult than in adults and modifications to surgical technique are required to minimize complications.

P. Kim, MBBS (Hons), FRANZCO
Department of Ophthalmology,
Toronto Western Hospital, University of Toronto,
399 Bathurst Street, East Wing 6E 401, M5T 2S8
Toronto, ON, Canada
e-mail: peterkim76@gmail.com

D.S. Rootman, M.D., FRCSC (✉)
Department of Ophthalmology and Visual Sciences,
Toronto Western Hospital, University of Toronto,
399 Bathurst Street, East Wing 6E 401,
M5T 2S8 Toronto, ON, Canada
e-mail: d.rootman@utoronto.ca

T. Reinhard, F. Larkin (eds.), *Corneal Disease*,
DOI 10.1007/978-3-642-28747-3_7, © Springer-Verlag Berlin Heidelberg 2013

- Regular postoperative examinations are required and sutures are removed earlier following keratoplasty in infants.
- Early optical correction and aggressive amblyopia therapy are necessary to optimize visual outcomes.
- Glaucoma, immune rejection, and graft failure are important postoperative complications.

Introduction

Infant keratoplasty presents a unique set of issues and special challenges that are distinct from adult keratoplasty. The aim of penetrating keratoplasty in infants is to clear the visual axis to minimize deprivational amblyopia and thereby allow for functional visual development [11, 13]. The results of surgery have improved considerably since the 1960s due to advancements in our understanding of the biology of the infant eye, improved microsurgical techniques and instruments, suture materials as well as improved postoperative management [3, 25, 45, 53]. The reported results of pediatric keratoplasty are generally poorer in infants and young children with higher graft failure rates when compared with adults [25, 51]. Nevertheless, many children can be greatly helped by the surgery with many developing useful, if not near normal, vision. Important considerations in infant keratoplasty include increased technical difficulties with surgery, more complex postoperative care, as well as higher graft failure rates.

Indications for Surgery

The causes of corneal opacity in infancy are categorized into congenital, acquired nontraumatic, and acquired traumatic groups [29, 45]. Congenital causes include Peters' anomaly, congenital glaucoma, dermoid, posterior polymorphous dystrophy, congenital hereditary endothelial dystrophy (CHED), congenital hereditary stromal dystrophy, sclerocornea, and metabolic disorders. Acquired nontraumatic causes include infectious keratitis (bacterial, viral, and fungal), interstitial keratitis, keratoconus, and exposure keratopathy. Penetrating and non-penetrating trauma of the cornea comprise the acquired traumatic causes. In developed countries, congenital causes of corneal opacities tend to predominate whilst in developing countries acquired traumatic and nontraumatic causes are more commonly encountered [1, 3, 19, 43, 49].

Visual Outcome

Studies have shown that early refractive correction and aggressive amblyopia therapy are critical for visual rehabilitation following pediatric penetrating keratoplasty [1, 16, 24]. Other important prognostic factors include significant postoperative astigmatism, strabismus, ocular comorbidities such as glaucoma and systemic comorbidities including developmental delay [11].

Visual prognosis appears to be closely related to underlying ocular pathology. In congenital opacities, eyes with isolated corneal opacity such as CHED, and Peters' anomaly type 1 have better visual outcomes and graft survival rates compared to eyes with associated anterior segment anomalies such as seen in advanced Peter's anomaly as well as sclerocornea [3, 26, 42, 52].

The visual outcomes reported in the published literature vary significantly and are not directly comparable due to study differences in underlying pathology, age distribution, postoperative care as well as follow-up duration [15, 24, 29, 38]. The indications for surgery vary between published studies with a high prevalence of CHED being reported in series from Saudi Arabia and Iran whilst infectious keratitis and trauma are important causes in studies from India [3, 26, 43, 49]. In the reported literature, acquired traumatic and nontraumatic indications for corneal transplantation have better rates of graft survival and visual outcomes compared to congenital indications [1, 3, 38].

Patient Selection

The decision to operate in infants with corneal opacity is often difficult. Surgery is considered if significant corneal opacification, either unilateral or bilateral, is present [11, 40]. Some surgeons do not operate on unilateral corneal opacities. However, we feel that the entire eye and patient should be considered. That is, eyes with isolated corneal opacity that are otherwise normal in terms of structure and size tend to have a good prognosis, and it is worthwhile to attempt corneal transplantation. On the other hand, bilateral cases with very complex anterior segment pathologies may not be amenable to surgery and have a high rate of complications such as retinal detachment. In these cases, it may be advisable to leave the child with the vision available, rather than risk total loss of the vision.

The main aim of surgery is to clear the visual axis and thereby promote functional visual development [11]. In the surgeon's decision-making process, the aims and risks of keratoplasty, ocular and systemic comorbidities as well as the ability of family members to comply with postoperative medications and follow-up visits must be considered.

For significant bilateral congenital corneal opacities, surgery is ideally performed within 3 months of life to minimize the risk of dense and irreversible amblyopia [11, 25]. In our center, we usually operate after the child is at least 1 month of age as this allows for some growth of the eye, making surgery somewhat easier as well as general anesthesia in these infants safer. The second eye can then be operated on 4–6 weeks later where sutures from the first operation may be removed [25]. This treatment strategy allows us to perform bilateral penetrating keratoplasty surgeries and removal of most sutures by 3 months of age. Interestingly, published studies so far have not proven better visual outcomes with earlier surgical intervention [3, 16, 26, 29, 52]. If there is marked asymmetry of the corneal opacification, it may be preferable in some situations to not operate and manage the less severely affected eye conservatively [21]. In cases with very poor prognosis secondary to very late presentation or advanced pathology, it may sometimes be preferable to offer no treatment, e.g., complex sclerocornea with associated severe anterior segment dysgenesis [25].

Realistic expectations by family members and the ability to commit to the required long-term postoperative care are prerequisites for surgery [21]. That is, penetrating keratoplasty will greatly impact all family members as frequent postoperative visits are required as well as imposing a significant financial burden [16, 44]. Multiple trips to the hospital for examinations and examinations under anesthesia (EUA) may be difficult or not possible if patients live far from the hospital center. Thus, the decision to operate as well as surgical timing must be individualized, taking into careful consideration the risks and benefits of surgery.

Summary for the Clinician

- The decision to operate must be individualized.
- Realistic expectations by family members, ability to administer postoperative medications as well as comply with follow-up visits are critical.

Patient Assessment

The preoperative assessment may be challenging and often requires an EUA. A careful history and thorough examination are essential as well as appropriate ancillary testing. A detailed history on presenting complaints, development milestones, gestational age and birth weight, medication use, and maternal history (including pregnancy and birth) provides important information for the clinician [11]. The onset and progression of corneal opacity is particularly important as this has important prognostic implications. That is, acquired opacities generally have better visual outcomes compared to congenital opacities [15, 29]. It is prudent to enquire into any family history of ocular anomalies such as posterior polymorphous dystrophy, anterior segment dysgenesis, glaucoma, etc.

On examination, careful assessment of the child's visual behavior including fixation pattern is important. The presence or absence of nystagmus or a relative afferent pupillary defect should be noted. A portable slit lamp is an essential tool to adequately examine the child's anterior segment. The examiner may be able to adequately assess the anterior segment by holding the bundled infant up to the slit lamp. Important features to note include an assessment of the eyelids as well as thorough examination of the cornea including corneal diameter, opacity (extent and severity), and vascularization. The anterior chamber anatomy including iris, angle, and lens anomalies should be noted. Looking at the quality of the red reflex with the direct ophthalmoscope will indicate the visual significance of the opacity. Intraocular pressure (IOP) can be measured by an electronic applanation tonometers, e.g., Tono-Pen® (Reichert, Depew, NY). A dilated fundus examination is required to exclude the presence of ocular comorbidities such as optic nerve, macular, and retinal pathology. If precluded by the opacity, a B scan ultrasound may be useful to ensure retinal attachment. A cycloplegic refraction should also be performed if possible. An EUA is usually required to thoroughly assess the infants' ocular pathology.

The presence of significant comorbidities may preclude surgery and referral to a pediatrician may occasionally be necessary.

Summary for the Clinician

- A comprehensive history and clinical examination often gives clues to the underlying etiology and visual prognosis.
- An examination under anesthetic is often required for a thorough assessment.

Ancillary Testing

Ultrasound biomicroscopy (UBM) is a very useful tool as it allows for detailed visualization of the underlying anterior segment structures (Fig. 7.1) [29, 33]. It greatly assists in preoperative diagnosis and surgical planning in eyes with severe corneal opacity. An additional benefit is that the images obtained are often helpful in explaining to parents the infants' condition. In addition, a B-scan ultrasound may be performed to exclude posterior segment pathology and an A-scan can be performed to measure axial length (e.g., microphthalmia, buphthalmos). In some cases, electrophysiological testing with electroretinogram and/or visual evoked potential may be performed to determine the visual potential of the eye.

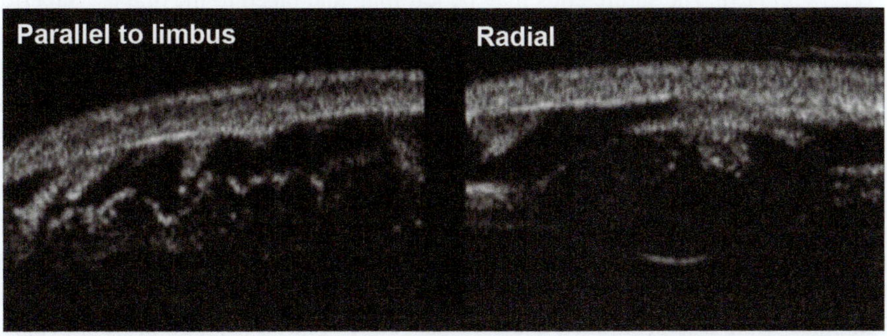

Fig. 7.1 UBM images taken parallel to the limbus shows extensive peripheral anterior synechiae. The image taken radially shows lenticulocorneal touch

Donor Tissue

Younger donor tissue with high endothelial cell counts is ideal but often not possible due to tissue availability. Infant donor tissue (<2 years old) is not recommended as the corneal tissue is thinner and therefore makes wound closure more difficult as well as the risk of progressive ectasia and steep corneal curvatures [28]. Death to preservation time, storage to use time, or method of storage has not been shown to have any effect on graft survival [48]. There is still controversy whether HLA matching has any benefits on immune allograft rejection and graft survival [22, 47]. However, ABO matching may have some benefit [47].

Intraoperative Considerations

Penetrating keratoplasty is performed under general anesthesia. The surgery is technically more difficult as the infant eye is smaller and the palpebral fissure is narrower. Occasionally, a lateral canthotomy may be required to improve surgical access.

Although similar to adult penetrating keratoplasty, certain important surgical modifications are required. A smaller sized graft is required, usually 6–7 mm, but occasionally smaller, to avoid sutures encroaching onto the limbus [40]. This will also keep the graft/host margin away from the limbus that may prevent peripheral anterior synechia from forming. Oversizing the donor tissue by 0.5–1.0 mm is recommended as this assists in wound closure as well as increasing anterior chamber depth [49]. The donor corneal button should be prepared prior to excising the host anterior chamber. An intracameral miotic should also be instilled if lensectomy is not planned to protect the crystalline lens.

The risk of lens extrusion and suprachoroidal hemorrhage is increased in infant keratoplasty secondary to decreased scleral rigidity and increased posterior vitreous pressure (Fig. 7.1) [11, 40]. It is important to use a Flieringa ring or an equivalent to stabilize the globe, taking care not to inadvertently perforate the thin infant sclera (Fig. 7.2) [13]. The suture ends may be left long and taped to the drapes. Superior and inferior rectus bridle sutures may offer additional control of the globe. Other techniques include the use of non-depolarizing muscle relaxants to eliminate the risk of extraocular muscle contraction during the surgical procedure; positioning the patient in a slight head down position; controlled hyperventilation; intravenous mannitol 20% (0.5–1.5 g/kg), and preoperative ocular massage [18, 36, 41].

As the infant cornea is thinner and more pliable than in adults, suturing and tissue apposition is more difficult [11]. Once the recipient corneal button has been excised, it is important to suture the donor button efficiently. Preplaced mattress bridge sutures may be placed before trephination and used to hold the donor cornea in place while it is positioned and cardinal sutures placed [37]. To prevent postoperative pupillary block, peripheral iridectomies (PIs) should be performed. In Peter's anomaly, where there may be preexisting iridocorneal adhesions, it is important to perform four PIs. In this circumstance, PAS are likely to form, and the PIs tend to

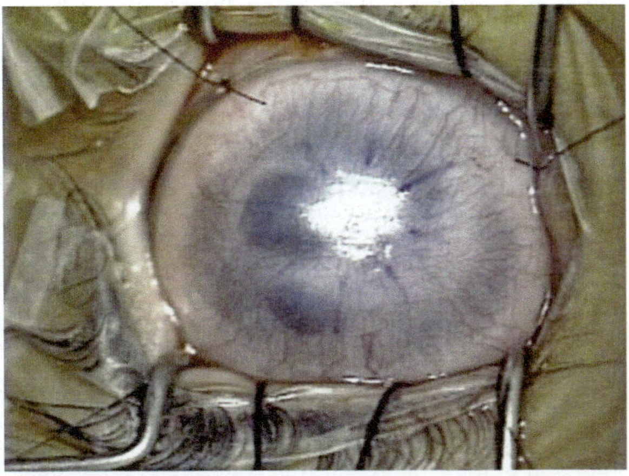

Fig. 7.2 This color photograph shows the operative set-up prior to performing penetrating keratoplasty. A Flieringa ring is placed and the suture ends left long and taped to the drapes. Using tape rather than hemostats greatly reduces the amount of hardware present close to the operative field. A superior and inferior rectus bridle suture is also present and the cornea has been marked with an 8-zone marker

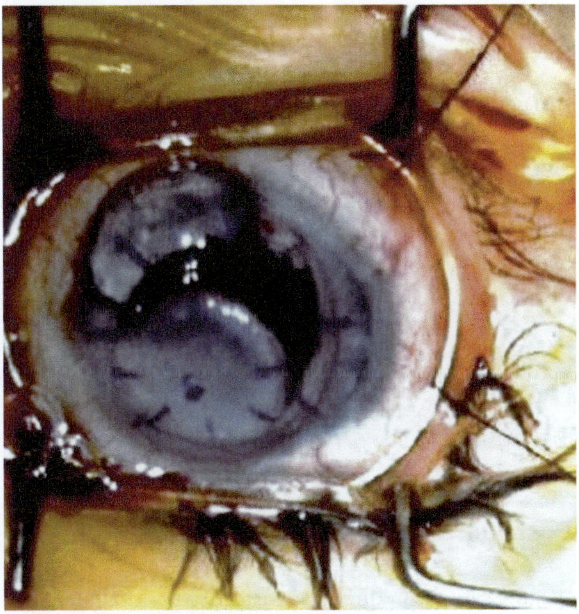

Fig. 7.3 Intraoperative lens extrusion following trephination of the recipient

limit progressive PAS in the postoperative period. Additionally, at the time of surgery, viscoelastic can be injected through a small paracentesis, and lyse any preexisting iridocorneal adhesions. This is much easier than trying to lyse the adhesions once the eye is "open sky" as the iris and/or lens often bulges forward (Fig. 7.3).

A watertight wound is critical at the conclusion of surgery and more than 16 sutures may be required to achieve this. The use of interrupted 10-0 nylon sutures is recommended. This ensures good wound closure with the thin infant recipient cornea. Additionally, if sutures loosen, break, or erode, they can be removed more easily without risking wound dehiscence, as is the case with a running suture technique. Subconjunctival antibiotics and steroids are administered and a firm pad and shield should be placed at the conclusion of surgery.

Concurrent Surgical Procedures

Concurrent procedures such as vitrectomy, synechiolysis, and lensectomy are known to be associated with poorer graft survival [1, 13, 24, 29, 45]. They may be planned or unplanned secondary to a surgical complication. When performing lensectomy concurrently with penetrating keratoplasty, it is often necessary to perform a posterior capsulotomy, anterior vitrectomy, and peripheral iridectomy. All vitreous in the anterior chamber should be removed with care to prevent vitreous adhering to the wound and iris. If possible, it has been the practice at our center to stage the cataract removal. In other words, if a cataract is present, or there is firm corneo-lenticular adhesion, the lens is removed whilst preserving the posterior capsule. Then at a later date, 2–4 weeks after the transplantation, a pars plicata, closed capsulectomy can be performed. We believe this approach is safer for the patient and allows for a more thorough removal of the vitreous in a closed ocular setting.

Summary for the Clinician

- Penetrating keratoplasty in infants is more difficult secondary to decreased scleral rigidity and increased posterior vitreous pressure and modifications to surgical technique are required.
- Interrupted 10-0 nylon sutures are recommended to reduce the risk of wound dehiscence.
- Concurrent procedures, whether planned or unplanned, are associated with reduced graft survival.

Postoperative Considerations

Postoperative care in infants is different to adults and is often challenging. A protective shield is essential and in some circumstances, arm restraints or splints may be necessary. However, young infants rarely generate much force, so self-injury is uncommon. Initially, topical antibiotics, corticosteroids, and cycloplegics are started and parents must understand the importance of compliance with medications. Corticosteroids are used at a higher dose and tapered more slowly than in adults as the inflammatory response is markedly greater in the pediatric age group. Cosar et al. [14] described the addition of topical cyclosporine 2% to topical corticosteroids in pediatric keratoplasty and found a reduced immune rejection rate compared with using corticosteroids alone. Family members should be instructed not to force the eye open when instilling drops as excessive force may result in inadvertent wound rupture. An alternative is for drops to be instilled in the nasal corner of the eye, and as the child blinks, the medication will reach the anterior segment.

Infants can usually be examined with a portable slit lamp whilst sitting on the parents' lap or whilst feeding. Otherwise they may be wrapped with a blanket and restrained, with or without the use of a lid speculum. Nonetheless, it is best to try and sneak up on a calm infant. One needs to only inspect for graft clarity, integrity of the wound, loose sutures, and presence of an anterior chamber. If there is poor cooperation, an EUA may need to be performed. Regular follow-up examinations are required as infants are unable to communicate their symptoms.

In the initial postoperative period, it is important to ensure that the wound is watertight, the anterior chamber is formed, and the IOP is within normal range. In the first 1–2 weeks, the infant is monitored closely until the ocular surface is fully epithelialized as a persistent epithelial defect is a risk factor for microbial keratitis [50].

Suture Management

In infants, sutures may be removed as early as 4 weeks due to their faster wound healing [24, 29]. The infant needs to be monitored at least weekly until all sutures are removed. Suture removal is incrementally delayed with increasing age of the child and must be balanced against the risk of graft dehiscence. Any loose, eroded, or broken sutures should be removed promptly to avoid suture-related infection and neovascularization. The precise timing in ceasing topical antibiotics varies by practice but may be discontinued a month or so after all sutures have been removed [50].

Optical Correction and Amblyopia Therapy

Amblyopia is a unique and important consideration following penetrating keratoplasty in infants and young children [21, 29]. It is a major factor limiting postoperative visual outcome despite surgical success. Joint management with a pediatric ophthalmologist is helpful for early refractive correction and aggressive amblyopia therapy [24]. Regular cycloplegic refractions are required following surgery and performed as soon as possible after surgery. Although contact lenses are associated with an increased risk of corneal neovascularization and infectious keratitis, they may be very useful if high anisometropia is present [10]. Parents should also be informed that regular prescription changes may be required postoperatively.

Summary for the Clinician

- Compliance with postoperative care including the proper administration of eye drops is crucial for graft survival.
- Regular postoperative follow-up including EUAs are required as infants are unable to communicate their symptoms.
- Sutures can be removed significantly earlier in infants due to their faster wound healing.
- Optical correction and amblyopia therapy should be initiated early to optimize visual outcomes.

Postoperative Complications

Glaucoma

Glaucoma is a frequent complicating factor in infants who have had penetrating keratoplasty surgery. The etiological mechanisms are diverse and include steroid-induced glaucoma, associated anterior segment dysgenesis, persistent anterior chamber inflammation, peripheral anterior synechiae, and surgically induced trabecular meshwork collapse http://www.expertconsultbook.com/expertconsult/b/linkTo?type=bookPage&isbn=978-0-323-06387-6&eid=4-u1.0-B978-0-323-06387-6..00132-X--bib76&appID=NGE [29, 35]. Glaucoma is associated with reduced allograft survival as well as causing irreversible optic nerve damage [3, 13, 16, 43, 45, 53].

Initial management includes topical glaucoma medications such as beta-adrenergic antagonists, carbonic anhydrase inhibitors, and prostaglandin analogs [29, 34]. Selective α-adrenergic agonists should be avoided as they may cause central nervous system depression in infants and young children [9]. It is important to regularly monitor infants for side effects from topical glaucoma medications. In patients where medical therapy does not adequately control IOP or is not tolerated, surgical intervention may be required. Surgical options include goniotomy, trabeculectomy with or without an anti-fibrotic agent, glaucoma drainage tube insertion, and cyclodestructive procedures [7, 25]. Occasionally, concurrent management of glaucoma and corneal opacification is required. The optimal timing and sequence of penetrating keratoplasty and glaucoma filtration procedures (trabeculectomy or tube) is still unclear [3, 4, 29]. Whenever possible, it is best to control the IOP prior to performing the corneal transplant as uncontrolled IOP may deleteriously affect the graft.

Graft Rejection

Immune rejection should be suspected in a cloudy allograft that was previously clear, particularly if associated with anterior chamber inflammation [45]. The classic signs of keratic precipitates or a Khoudadoust (rejection) line is less commonly

Table 7.1 Risk factors for graft failure [1, 3, 6, 11, 13, 16, 17, 24, 25, 29, 30, 38, 43, 45, 50, 52, 53]

1. Younger age
2. Congenital corneal opacities (cf. acquired causes)
3. Disease severity
4. Associated anterior segment anomalies (e.g., anterior synechiae)
5. Cornea vascularization
6. Concurrent surgical procedures (including lensectomy and anterior vitrectomy)
7. Regrafting
8. Donor corneal size
9. Postoperative complications
Persistent epithelial defects
Allograft rejection
Infectious keratitis
Retinal detachment
Glaucoma

seen in the pediatric age group [29, 44]. Most commonly, the patients present with diffuse epithelial edema of the corneal graft. Initial treatment consists of intensive topical corticosteroids such as dexamethasone 0.1% or prednisolone acetate 1% hourly that is titrated to treatment response. Topical cyclosporine may also have a role in the prevention of immune graft rejection in pediatric keratoplasty [14]. In recalcitrant cases, oral corticosteroids may be needed at a dosage of approximately 1 mg/kg/day.

Graft Failure

Allograft failure occurs most commonly within the first postoperative year and infants should be closely monitored during this period [3, 45]. The risk factors for graft failure are shown in Table 7.1. Repeat penetrating keratoplasty in infants is associated with a higher graft failure rate [16, 45]. In patients with possible immune rejection, a course of intensive topical steroids should be given. A regraft may be considered if the cornea fails to clear and the eye has been quiescent for at least 3 months.

Summary for the Clinician

- Glaucoma frequently complicates infant keratoplasty and should be managed appropriately as it is associated with increased risk of graft failure.
- Immune rejection and allograft failure are important postoperative complications of infant keratoplasty.

Alternatives to Penetrating Keratoplasty

It is important to consider alternatives to penetrating keratoplasty, particular those techniques that are less invasive but nevertheless effective [5, 8, 12, 20, 27]. For example, in some infants with a clear peripheral cornea and crystalline lens, an optical iridectomy may result in an acceptable visual outcome [46]. This is an effective surgical intervention, particularly if follow-up is likely to be difficult or unreliable, and may be the safer option in some cases [25, 29, 46].

Rotational autografts may be suitable in selected cases where a corneal opacity involving the pupillary area is rotated to leave a clear central visual axis [2, 31, 39].

In adults, lamellar techniques are now preferred over penetrating keratoplasty to selectively replace diseased tissue, thereby leaving healthy tissue untouched. For instance, endothelial keratoplasty is currently the preferred surgical technique for isolated endothelial disease such as Fuchs' endothelial keratoplasty and pseudophakic bullous keratopathy. The advantages of Descemet stripping endothelial keratoplasty (DSEK) over PK are numerous and include faster visual rehabilitation, less induced refractive error, a tectonically stronger eye, and less suture-related complications [12]. There have been a few case reports of successful DSEK in children with CHED [20, 27].

DSEK surgery is also technically more challenging in the pediatric age group due to their smaller anterior chamber dimensions and risk of cataract formation if iatrogenic damage to the crystalline lens occurs [12]. Furthermore, there is more difficult postoperative management in children secondary to compliance issues with posturing, etc. Nevertheless, DSEK may be an option for a selected group of patients, that is, those children with isolated endothelial disease [20, 27].

Similarly, deep anterior lamellar keratoplasty (DALK) may be preferred to PK in children with isolated stromal pathology, e.g., corneal scarring secondary to infectious keratitis, mucopolysaccharides, central dermoids, and keratoconus [23]. DALK is technically more challenging but is advantageous as it avoids an "open sky" procedure and essentially eliminates the risk of lens extrusion or suprachoroidal hemorrhage. There are different surgical techniques of performing DALK and include manual deep lamellar dissection, "big-bubble," and viscodissection.

The Boston keratoprosthesis has been performed in pediatric patients as an alternative to penetrating keratoplasty. The advantages include rapid visual rehabilitation, elimination of allograft rejection, and earlier initiation of amblyopia therapy [5]. It may have a role in children with poor prognosis for PK such as multiple allograft failures secondary to immune rejection [5, 8, 12]. However, disadvantages include the need for a bandage contact lens, difficulty in monitoring intraocular pressure as well as the indefinite use of antibiotics [32]. Complications include retroprosthetic membrane, stromal thinning or melting, implant extrusion, sterile vitritis, and infectious endophthalmitis [32]. The long-term complications are of particular concern as these patients will have their prosthesis for a very long duration.

Summary for the Clinician

- An optical iridectomy is minimally invasive and may result in a good visual outcome in selected cases.
- Lamellar surgery including DSEK and DALK as well as the Boston keratoprosthesis has been performed successfully in pediatric patients.

Conclusion

Infant keratoplasty is challenging in many ways. Careful patient selection, meticulous preoperative planning and surgical technique, early refractive correction, and amblyopia therapy as well as regular follow-up are necessary to achieve best visual outcomes. This requires a team approach with close collaboration between the corneal surgeon, pediatric ophthalmologist, support staff as well as family members. The impact of achieving functional vision for children with severe corneal opacity cannot be overemphasized. It is associated with significant improvements in behavior, communication, and ambulation, as well as having tremendous benefits for the family members.

Conflict of Interest None of the authors have any financial/conflicting interests to disclose.

References

1. Aasuri MK, Garg P, Gokhle N et al (2000) Penetrating keratoplasty in children. Cornea 19:140–144
2. Afshari NA, Duncan SM, Tanhehco TY et al (2006) Optimal size and location for corneal rotational autografts. Arch Ophthalmol 124:410–413
3. Al-Ghamdi A, Al-Rajhi A, Wagoner MD (2007) Primary pediatric keratoplasty: indications, graft survival and visual outcome. JAAPOS 11:41–47
4. Al-Torbak AA (2004) Outcome of combined Ahmed glaucoma valve implant and penetrating keratoplasty in refractory congenital glaucoma with corneal opacity. Cornea 23:554–559
5. Aquavella JV (2008) Pediatric keratoplasties: a new surgical approach. Ann Ophthalmol 40:64–67
6. Beauchamp GR (1979) Pediatric keratoplasty: problems in management. J Pediatr Ophthalmol Strabismus 16:388–394
7. Beck AD (2001) Diagnosis and management of pediatric glaucoma. Ophthalmol Clin North Am 14:501–512
8. Botelho PJ, Congdon NG, Handa JT et al (2006) Keratoprosthesis in high-risk pediatric corneal transplantation: first 2 cases. Arch Ophthalmol 124:1356–1357
9. Bowman RJC, Cope J, Nischal KK (2004) Ocular and systemic side effects of brimonidine 0.2% eye drops in children. Eye 18:24–26
10. Calhoun J (1991) Cataracts and lens anomalies in children. In: Nelson LB, Calhoun JH, Harley RD (eds) Pediatric ophthalmology. WB Saunders, Philadelphia
11. Chan AS, Colby K (2008) Update on pediatric keratoplasty. Int Ophthalmol Clin 48:25–33
12. Colby K (2008) Changing times for pediatric keratoplasty. JAAPOS 12:223–224

13. Comer RM, Sheraz MD, O'Keefe M (2001) Penetrating keratoplasty in infants. JAAPOS 5:285–290
14. Cosar CB, Laibson LP, Cohen EJ et al (2003) Topical cyclosporine in pediatric keratoplasty. Eye Contact Lens 29:103–107
15. Cowden JW (1990) Penetrating keratoplasty in infants and children. Ophthalmology 97: 324–328
16. Dana MR, Moyes AL, Gomes JA et al (1995) The indications for and outcome in pediatric keratoplasty. A multicenter study. Ophthalmology 102:1129–1138
17. Dana MR, Schaumberg DA, Moyes AL et al (1995) Outcome of penetrating keratoplasty after ocular trauma in children. Arch Ophthalmol 113:1503–1507
18. Duncalf D, Weitzner SW (1963) Ventilation and hypercapnea on intraocular pressure during anaesthesia. Anaesthesia and Analgesia 42:232–237
19. Erlich C, Rootman DS, Morin J (1991) Corneal transplantation in infants, children and young adults: experience of the Toronto Hospital for Sick Children. 1979–88. Can J Ophthalmol 26: 206–210
20. Fernandez MM, Buckley EG, Afshari NA (2008) Descemet stripping automated endothelial keratoplasty in a child. JAAPOS 12:314–316
21. Gloor P (2005) Pediatric penetrating keratoplasty. In: Krachmer JH, Mannis MJ, Holland EJ (eds) Cornea. Elsevier, Philadelphia, pp 1591–1618
22. Gore SM, Vail A, Bradley VA et al (1995) HLA-DR matching in corneal transplantation. Systematic review of published evidence Corneal Tranplant Follow-up Study Collaborators. Transplantation 60:1033–1039
23. Harding SA, Nischal KK, Upponi-Patil A et al (2010) Indications and outcomes of deep anterior lamellar keratoplasty in children. Ophthalmology 117:2191–2195
24. Huang PT (2007) Penetrating keratoplasty in infants and children. JAAPOS 11:5–6
25. Hwang DG, Hwang PH (1991) Pediatric penetrating keratoplasty. Semin Ophthalmol 6:212–218
26. Javadi MA, Baradaran-Rafli AR, Zamani M et al (2003) Penetrating keratoplasty in young children with congential hereditary endothelial dystrophy. Cornea 22:420–423
27. Jeng BH, Marcotty A, Traboulsi E (2008) Descemet stripping automated endothelial keratoplasty in a 2-year-old child. JAAPOS 12:317–318
28. Koenig SB, Graul E, Kaufman E (1982) Ocular refraction after penetrating keratoplasty with infant donor corneas. Am J Ophthalmol 94:534–539
29. Lee OA, Lenhart PD, Holland EJ (2011) Pediatric Penetrating Keratoplasty. In: Krachmer JH, Mannis MJ, Holland EJ (eds) Cornea: fundamentals, diagnosis and management, 3rd edn. Mosby, Elsevier Inc., New York, pp 1455–1472
30. McClellan K, Lai T, Grigg J et al (2003) Penetrating keratoplasty in children: visual and graft outcome. Br J Ophthalmol 87:1212–1214
31. Murthy S, Bansal AK, Sridahr MS (2001) Ipsilateral rotational autokeratoplasty: an alternative to penetrating keratoplasty in nonprogressive central corneal scars. Cornea 20:455–457
32. Nallasamy S, Colby K (2010) Keratoprosthesis: procedure of choice for corneal opacities in children? Semin Ophthalmol 25:244–248
33. Nischal KK, Naor J, Jay V et al (2002) Clinicopathological correlation of congential corneal opacification using ultrasound biomicroscopy. Br J Ophthalmol 86:62–69
34. Olson RJ, Bromberg BB, Zimmerman TJ (1979) Apneic spells associated with timolol therapy in a neonate. Am J Ophthalmol 88:120–122
35. Olson RJ, Kaufman HE (1977) A mathematical description of causative factors and prevention of elevated intraocular pressure after keratoplasty. Invest Ophthalmol Vis Sci 16:1085–1092
36. Ozcan MS, Praetel C, Bhatti MT et al (2004) The effect of body inclination during prone positioning on intraocular pressure in awake volunteers: a comparison of two operating tables. Anesth Analg 99:1152–1158
37. Parrish CM, Faris DA, O'Day DM (1988) Mattress bridge sutures for graft fixation in pediatric keratoplasty: new use of an old technique. Ophthalmic Surg 19:795–798
38. Patel HY, Ormonde S, Brookes NH et al (2005) The indications and outcome of paediatric corneal transplantation in New Zealand: 1991–2003. Br J Ophthalmol 89:404–408

39. Rao SK, Lam DSC (2008) Calculating graft size and position in rotational corneal autografting: a simplified approach. Indian J Ophthalmol 56:233–235
40. Reidy J (2001) Penetrating keratoplasty in infancy and early childhood. Curr Opin Ophthalmol 12:258–261
41. Robbins R, Blumenthal M, Galin MA (1970) Reduction of vitreous weight by ocular massage. Am J Ophthalmol 69:603–607
42. Schaumberg DA, Moyes AL, Gomes JA et al (1999) Corneal transplantation in young children with congenital hereditary endothelial dystrophy. Multicenter Pediatric Keratoplasty Study. Am J Ophthalmol 127:373–378
43. Sharma N, Prakash G, Titiyal JS et al (2007) Pediatric keratoplasty in India: indications and outcomes. Cornea 26:810–813
44. Stulting RD (1993) Penetrating keratoplasty in children. In: Brightbill F (ed) Corneal surgery: theory, technique, and tissue. Mosby, St. Louis
45. Stulting RD, Sumers KD, Cavanagh HD et al (1984) Penetrating keratoplasty in children. Ophthalmology 91:1222–1230
46. Sundaresh K, Jethani J, Vijayalakshmi P (2008) Optical iridectomy in children with corneal opacities. JAAPOS 12:163–165
47. The Collaborative Corneal Transplantation Studies Research Group (1992) The collaborative corneal transplantation studies (CCTS). Effectiveness of histocompatibility matching in high-risk corneal transplantation. Arch Ophthalmol 110:1392–1403
48. Vail A, Gore SM, Bradley BA et al (1994) Influence of donor and histocompatibility factors on corneal graft outcome. Transplantation 58:1210–1216
49. Vajpayee RB, Ramu M, Panda A et al (1999) Oversized grafts in children. Ophthalmology 106:829–832
50. Wagoner MD, Al-Ghamdi AH, Al-Rajhi AA (2007) Bacterial keratitis after primary pediatric penetrating keratoplasty. Am J Ophthalmol 143:1045–1047
51. Williams KA, Roder D, Esterman AEA (1992) Factors predictive of corneal graft survival: report from the Australian Corneal Graft Registry. Ophthalmology 99:403–414
52. Yang LL, Lambert SR (2009) Long-term visual outcome of penetrating keratoplasty in infants and children with Peters anomaly. JAAPOS 13:175–180
53. Zaidman GW, Flanagan JK, Furey CC (2007) Long-term visual prognosis in children after corneal transplant surgery for Peters anomaly type 1. Am J Ophthalmol 144:104–108

Index

T. Reinhard, F. Larkin (eds.), *Corneal Disease*,
DOI 10.1007/978-3-642-28747-3, © Springer-Verlag Berlin Heidelberg 2013

GPSR Compliance

The European Union's (EU) General Product Safety Regulation (GPSR) is a set of rules that requires consumer products to be safe and our obligations to ensure this.

If you have any concerns about our products, you can contact us on ProductSafety@springernature.com

In case Publisher is established outside the EU, the EU authorized representative is:

Springer Nature Customer Service Center GmbH
Europaplatz 3
69115 Heidelberg, Germany

Batch number: 10584666

Printed by Printforce, the Netherlands